connections

Animal Assisted Therapy
For Alzheimer's Disease
And Related Dementias

By Pam Osbourne

Copyright Notices

International Standard Book Number (ISBN)
978-0-9993761-0-2

Legal Notices

While all attempts have been made to give readers accurate cutting edge information, neither the author nor the publisher assumes any responsibility for errors, omissions or contradictory interpretations of the subject matter herein.

The purchaser or reader of this publication assumes responsibility for the use of these materials and information. Adherence to all applicable laws and regulations, federal, state, and local, governing professional licensing, business practices, advertising and all other aspects of doing business in the United States or any other jurisdiction is the sole responsibility of the purchaser or reader. PYOW Publishing assumes no responsibility or liability whatsoever on behalf of any purchaser or reader.

Dedication

For my mom and dad,

Irene and John Skwira

Mom, who kept on trying,

and

Dad, who never left her side

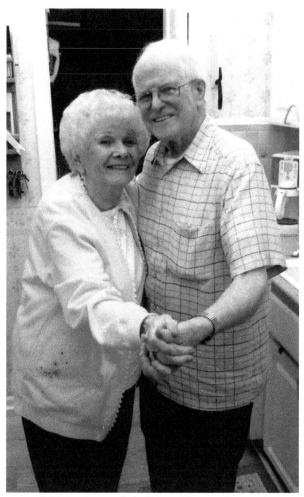

Still dancing on their 65ᵗʰ wedding anniversary!

TABLE OF CONTENTS

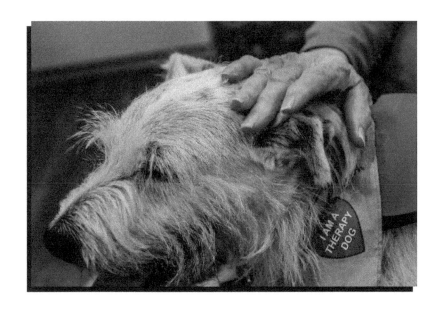

Introduction

Being in the presence of animals helps people with Alzheimer's Disease and Related Dementias (ADRD)* feel connected, oriented, and less alienated from the world. Interacting (petting, talking, feeding, etc.) with animals causes a healthy connection that has been scientifically proven to be therapeutic.

By their very nature people have a deep seated need to be connected to themselves, other people, other forms of life, and the world around them. When this connection is made, people feel oriented. They feel at home with themselves and the world in which they find themselves.

Connecting the experiential dots is a basic function of the human mind. Doing so enables people to develop an orientation to life, an understanding of life and a sense of direction, purpose and continuity that allows them to function and to interact with themselves and others in a meaningful way, a way that makes sense.

Dementia causes a person's connections to disintegrate. It causes a person to feel disoriented and alienated from themselves and the world in which they find themselves.

It is a disease that tends to reduce and dismantle the dot connecting process. It happens gradually, over time. Generally speaking it happens with older folks who find themselves becoming forgetful, losing their orientation, and becoming unable to understand themselves and others in a meaningful way.

My own personal experience happened when my mom was diagnosed with dementia at about age 87. During the last six years of her life, the time I spent with Mom was always enhanced by connections.

With music, we connected by listening, singing, and dancing together. The old standards and some polka music prompted us to burst into song at times and even get up to dance a few steps. We were the polka queens.

We connected with food. We could still spend a day together making home-made pierogi, or just go out for a hot fudge sundae, her favorite.

But, the best connector was my dog, Rufus. Rufus and I are a trained registered therapy team. For over ten years Rufus has enriched the lives of countless people (who have, in turn, enriched ours), young and old, by making someone's ordinary day extraordinary. He has that same effect on our family, and he had it on my mom and dad.

Whether you are a health care professional, Animal Assisted Therapy team, family member, friend, or caregiver, there are a variety of Animal Assisted Therapy activities that will have a very positive effect. Activities range from assisting in simple everyday tasks such as eating and dressing, to physical therapy, functional exercises, to just having a good visit.

The mere presence of a dog will provide a calming connection. The activities included in this book often make an astounding difference to those with ADRD. My experience with Animal Assisted Therapy and my mom demonstrates another way to maintain and encourage meaningful connections.

This book is intended to be a user friendly guide for Animal Assisted Therapy teams, healthcare professionals, or family members and friends, by first providing some essential background information, then suggested activities.

---

*Alzheimer's Disease is the most common form of dementia. Dementia is a general term used to describe loss of memory and other intellectual abilities that interfere with daily life. A diagnosis is based on a doctor's best judgement combined with tests and observations.

There is a growing number of related dementias. Among them are: Vascular dementia, Mixed dementia, Parkinson's disease, Dementia with Lewy bodies, Huntington's disease, Pick's disease, Normal Pressure Hydrocephalus (NPH), Creutzfeldt-Jakob disease (CJD) and dementia caused by physical injury to the brain. Still others are readily found on the Alzheimer's Association's website www.alz.org, and related publications.

connections

PART I

Enter Alzheimer's Disease
My Personal Experience

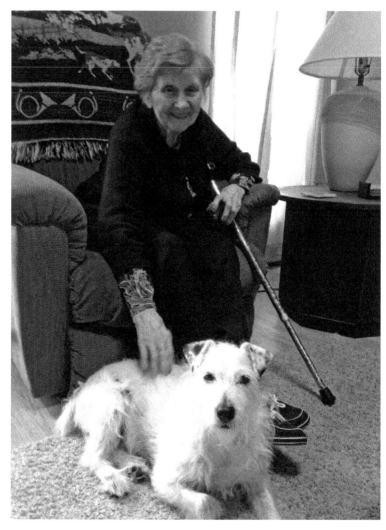

Mom reaches for Rufus, Rufus reaches Mom…
a connection is made.

1

Irene, My Mom

I lost my mom long before she ever died. Our journey (and it IS a journey) with ADRD began in June of 2010. Mom was 87, and by all accounts was that vibrant, active "blondie" that we always knew. She had her hair "done" every week, played bingo, and still danced a mean polka.

Since we all lived in the suburban Chicago area, we were able to visit Mom and Dad regularly, gathering for holidays and other occasions. We were a typical family, with parents who had been married for 67 years with two children (my brother, Al, and myself), three grandchildren (Bonnie, Kiki, and Cody), and two great-grandchildren (Alex and Austin). Life seemed "normal."

At 87, Mom had her share of health issues. Doctor visits became more frequent. In our desire to help get to the bottom of some of her issues, we began to accompany both Mom and Dad on their doctor visits. By having more frequent contact, my brother and I began to notice that things were not quite as normal as we believed.

The journey begins

Mom seemed to be forgetting things frequently, so when we mentioned it to her doctor she was referred to a neurologist. The CT scan she ordered revealed a normal brain for a woman her age. We were encouraged by that.

As for me, I fell into a false sense of security that things were okay. Even though Mom only scored 10 out of 30 on the "memory test," what could possibly be wrong? As we sat in that doctor's office while Mom struggled for answers

> **Alzheimer's Disease** is NOT a normal part of aging, but is much more serious, worsening over time, with *no known cure*. Fifty to seventy percent of dementia cases fall into this category.

to the doctor's questions, the anguish on Dad's face was almost too much to bear. Because of these "slight" memory issues, Mom was given Aricept, a well-known drug in the treatment of dementia. It is important to know that these drugs are not a "cure" for ADRD.

> **Warning sign: Memory changes that disrupt daily life**
> When I would call Mom, she would always tell me that she hadn't heard from me in a long time, even if I had just talked with her that morning. When I'd tell her things about the kids or other family members, she would say, "you never told me that." At the time, I thought she was just complaining too much. I didn't realize that she really didn't remember that she had spoken with me an hour before, or the day before.

At that point, we were just beginning to learn that there is no known cure for what we would eventually come to refer to as "this insidious disease." I'm not sure that we noticed a significant difference in her memory after taking the drug, but at the time we also didn't know that she wasn't going to get better. These drugs simply "fend off" deterioration at best.

When Mom was sick for two weeks with vomiting and diarrhea, to the point that she couldn't even dress herself without assistance, the doctor was reluctant to admit her to the hospital. She instead recommended that Mom drink more liquids, and told her to be sure to eat better. In response to that, we took action, ordered "Meals on Wheels" and increased our visits with them. Unfortunately, most of the meals ended up stacked in their refrigerator unopened.

The "new normal"

Finally, Mom was admitted to the hospital, but her visit revealed no conclusive outcomes. From there, she was sent to rehab for five days, with no good results there either. Upon returning home, she was visited by a home health nurse, who reviewed her medications and asked why she was on Aricept (on the maximum dosage) because the side effects could be causing some of the issues that landed her in the hospital.

The nurse gave us some good information, but her best piece of advice was that we were now experiencing the "new normal" in our family. That phrase sustained and comforted me through the coming years. It was the realization that "normal" has a variety of meanings.

At that point, we were just learning about the side effects and interactions of the medications both Mom and Dad were taking. Immediately, we asked to stop the Aricept, and weaned her off of it (Something else I didn't know about...that you just don't stop taking these drugs "cold turkey"). Once she was weaned off Aricept, though, she seemed more confused, and became almost uncommunicative.

I would take her for drives and talk about the weather, shopping, or family news, and she would be almost unresponsive, in contrast to her chatty self. That was when we learned that there are a variety of medications available for treating ADRD.

It seems that there is a fair amount of "trial and error" to find the best medications for each individual. So, the doctor started her on Namenda, and she seemed to be back to her "new normal" self now without the extreme side effects.

> **Warning sign:** Difficulty completing familiar tasks at home, at work or at leisure
>
> We called Mom "Mrs. Clean," but now Dad did most of the cleaning. Mom stopped shopping and preparing meals. She was the photo keeper in our family, so I asked if she would put together photo books for Al and me. But, she couldn't sort or organize them. She just got frustrated with the project, and started to throw pictures away, because she said she didn't know these people anyway. That was when all the family photos moved to my house.

Bingo!

Social contacts for Mom, other than family, became a trip to the beauty shop once a week, and bingo. During this time, I received a phone call from one of her bingo buddies who said she was worried about Mom, because she was having a hard time playing bingo. What? Mom was a woman who had a history of playing 20 cards at a time.

So, I decided to take her to bingo to see for myself. I was horrified to find that her friends were not only setting up her cards, but "spotting" the numbers for her. At times she didn't even know when games were ending or beginning. She told me that she was having difficulty hearing the numbers called and that was why she couldn't play. That, I think, was her last bingo night. She actually didn't want to go after that, even though I said I would go with her and help.

> **Warning sign:**
> **Withdrawal from work or social activities**
> Mom didn't want to go to the beauty shop or Bingo.

Isolation seemed to increase for both Mom and Dad. She also started to rely on Dad to speak for her. When asked a question, she looked to him to answer for her. Prior to this, Mom was the one who took charge of everything, and did the talking (and lots of it!). Now Dad was in charge of virtually everything in the house, from cleaning to preparing meals, doing the laundry and monitoring their medications.

> **Warning sign:**
> **Challenges in planning or solving problems**
> Mom was an expert at knitting and crocheting. She was still able to pick up the knitting needles or crochet hook without missing a beat, and start right in. The problem was she no longer could follow directions or a pattern. She made a lot of circles with her crochet hook, and the knitting produced uneven rows. She didn't know when to begin or end a row.

The home health nurse had set up some physical therapy at home. One of the best therapy professionals we worked with was a speech pathologist. He focused on her verbal skills, encouraging her to speak. He was also the one who recommended that I make a photo book of people in her life, identifying each person.

We wrote down Mom's name and address, so every day we could talk about it with her. We made sure to write events in their calendar so she could look at it every day, and see what day/date it was. We could talk about daily activities. He encouraged us to interact with her in any way that would encourage her to speak.

He recommended word search books as good "brain games" but she had absolutely no interest in them. She never really did anything like that before, so she wasn't about to start now. The word find books lay untouched. Instead, I encouraged her to pick up her knitting and crocheting again. She had made so many sweaters, afghans, etc. over the years with complicated patterns that challenged her brain, but at that point she was only able to do some of the simpler projects, with guidance.

I was never at her level of expertise when it came to knitting and crocheting, but I knew enough that I could work alongside her, and I could read the directions, step by step. We made lots of crocheted hangers and knitted dishcloths! It was such a great activity to do together. With her favorite polka music in the background, we had many pleasant afternoons.

More confusion

About that time, her teeth went missing. It was only her "uppers" but she needed them! We immediately went to the dentist, and within a month (a long time without teeth!) she had a new set, *plus* a spare. But, then her glasses went missing. At least she was able to get new glasses within a few days. The lost teeth and glasses never did surface.

> **Warning sign:**
> **Misplacing things and losing the ability to retrace steps**
> Her teeth and glasses were misplaced on a regular basis. At times she wasn't even aware whether or not she was wearing glasses.

She didn't seem to know that her home was actually her home. She would say that "this place has some really nice furniture." By then we had learned to go along with her conversation, so we would agree with her. In those early days, I always hoped that she would realize where she was. But that never happened. If we told her this was her furniture, she would respond with, "oh, really?" Sometimes she wouldn't recognize the furniture, and frequently accused my brother of selling it all.

Further evaluation needed

We arranged an appointment with a neuro psychologist for further evaluation. When he asked how long this had been going on, my brother and I said, "oh, probably a few months." The doctor shook his head and said that it had probably been going on for many years. I was sure taken aback. How could I have not noticed? To me, it was simply signs of growing old.

> **Warning sign: Confusion with time or place**
>
> She would say how much she liked the furniture in this place, even though it was her own home. She also would tell us that she didn't know where the bathroom was in this place.

His recommendation was that Mom needed care "24/7," and someone from the outside was needed to step in. Dad really did not agree that they needed help "24/7," or even needed any help at all. They were still living in their condominium, and he was in charge. However, we saw them struggling more and more.

Options

Al and I talked about options, none of which went over very well with my dad. We used the strategy of presenting two choices, then we'd say, "so which place would you like to visit and then consider a move?" Dad would say that they were choosing option number three, which was *their* choice to stay right where they were. My dad would have none of the other choices. "Those places were for *old* people." He did everything for Mom. It was an amazing act of love on his part.

They did agree to a two week "trial" stay at a senior community, The Meadows in Glen Ellyn, IL. While Dad didn't really like it, Mom seemed to enjoy it. To us, it seemed that the socialization perked her up a bit and motivated her to move a little more. In addition, they were closer to both Al and me, so we were able to visit them on a much more regular basis. However, they went back home after that stay and didn't take any more action in that direction.

A turning point

A couple of months later, Mom fell and broke her wrist. I think it was the event that made Dad realize he couldn't do it all. I lived 45 minutes away, and Al lived over an hour away from them. We needed them closer to at least one of us, so we could help. (Caregivers were out of the question. No "strangers" would be allowed in by Dad.) However, we also realized that Dad needed to be independent.

Timing is everything. About that time, I got an email about some special rates being offered at the Devonshire in Hoffman Estates, only about seven minutes from my brother. I called Dad, and said I'd pick up him and Mom and take them there for a look. Al met us there, and after the tour, I almost fell out of my chair when Dad pulled out his checkbook and said he would make a deposit on the place. That set the wheels in motion for the beginning of our peace of mind...or so I thought.

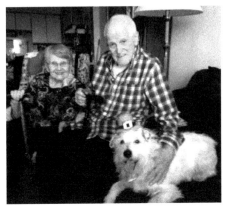

Reluctantly, they sold their condominium in Palos Heights. On St. Patrick's Day, 2011, they moved to the Devonshire, close to my brother, where they could have help, if needed.

Rufus helps celebrate their St. Patrick's Day move.

Road trip

The next November I took them on a trip to New York to visit with our dear cousins whom we had not seen for several years. Even though Mom and Dad were 89 years old, I felt it would be good for them to connect with some of their favorite people. What could be bad about this?

I would drive them cross country, a drive we made just about every other summer when I was growing up. It was so much easier back then with Dad driving, the wind blowing into our open car windows! I found that you can learn a lot about your aging parents when you're on such a long trip, being with them non-stop.

The preparation itself was daunting. At the time, Al was monitoring their medications, since he lived so close to them. He set up everything for me to take, and I felt confident that I was up for the task of making sure that they took everything they were supposed to, and on time. Piece of cake.

A few days before we were ready to leave, I brought out their suitcases. Mom and I packed hers, so it would be ready on the day of departure. I took them shopping, since Dad said he needed some warm shirts and sweatshirts. He said he could pack his own suitcase, so that was one less detail on my list.

> **Warning sign: Trouble understanding visual images and spatial relationships**
> Mom would often see double. She would point out things to me along the road that weren't there. When we got into the car, she would ask if her sister Rose was in the car, and if all the guys were in yet.

The day before departure, I went to their place and found that Mom had unpacked her suitcase, because she was looking for some shoes. She found a pair in the suitcase so she put them away, along with half of the other things in it. Undaunted, and calm with our "new normal," we re-packed, chose an outfit for her to wear the next day, and hung it on the door as a reminder. Dad said he would be packed by the morning.

I arrived the morning of the trip to find them still at breakfast, not ready to go, Mom's outfit still hanging on the door. The good news though, was that her suitcase was still packed, and Dad's was next to it. My plan was to make the drive in two days, (a one-day drive in the "old" days) knowing that we would have to make frequent stops along the way this time. It turned out that we stopped almost every hour, and all stops took a very long time. Just getting in and out of the car was challenging.

It was here that I really saw what Mom was going through. She had no sense of where she was, where she was going, or why she was there. I explained everything we were doing repeatedly. If I thought the lack of readiness for this trip was of concern, it was just the tip of the iceberg.

At the first rest stop, we walked into the building, and Mom immediately fell, despite the fact that she had her cane, and was holding on to me. I thought right then and there that our trip had ended without ever getting started. We were immediately surrounded by

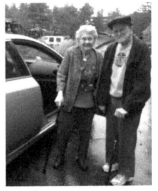

Rest stop number one

helpful folks, and once she stood up, she seemed okay. Fortunately, that wrist that she had broken months before was still intact.

My dad had always been great with directions and maps, so I thought that I'd have a great navigator on this trip. But, when I handed him the map, he said that he couldn't read it without a magnifying glass. So, at every rest stop (and there were many) I looked for a magnifier, but could never find one. It was at this point that I learned to actually use the GPS.

> **Warning sign: New problems with words in speaking or writing**
> Mom would start to say something, then not know how to finish it. When she would talk about someone, she couldn't remember who she was talking about. She began to speak less and less.

In the hotel room that first night, Dad emptied his pockets, and there among the change, gum, and other items, was his magnifier. The next revelation was when Dad opened his suitcase to get his pajamas. It was filled with socks and underwear, and none of the new clothes we had just bought. There was only one other shirt, and one pair of pants. I did see the logic of it in some respect. With Dad's congestive heart failure, and the drugs he was taking, he flew through underwear and socks.

We made our way to Syracuse the next day. At the rest stops, Mom needed constant monitoring and had trouble getting in and out of bathroom stalls. Then, once out, she did not know where to go. I stuck with her at all times, and worried about Dad, alone in the men's room. I had to ask several strange men to "please check on John in the bathroom."

None of this, though, overshadowed the fabulous time we had with our cousins in New York. I'm not sure what Mom remembered of them, but she sure seemed to enjoy herself. It was always a happy time with that "Buffalo Gang," and this was no exception. Mom and Dad just seemed so joyous when surrounded by them.

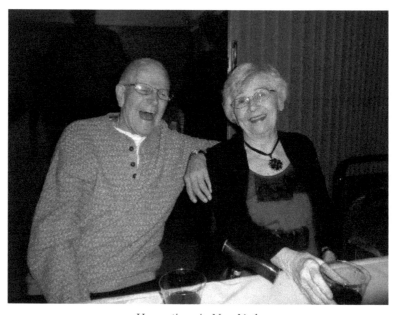

Happy times in New York

Once they were back at the Devonshire, I thought that they were at least in a safe place. We arranged for some other services, like medication reminders. We tried to set up other assistance for them, such as showers and assistance with dressing for Mom. But, Dad was opposed to it. He made that decision, and we lived with that "new normal."

For us, the important thing was monitoring the cocktail of medications they both needed. Also, it was imperative that my parents maintain their dignity and as much independence as possible. As long as no harm was occurring, we kept our distance. We really walked a fine line between helping them maintain their independence and safety.

Choose your battles

Mom needed more guidance with dressing, since she was unable to choose appropriate clothing for the weather. She also had begun sleeping in her clothes. She really wasn't aware that she needed to change clothes

I was there a couple times a week, or more, if doctor appointments or other activities were scheduled. Much of the time, Mom was wearing the same clothing she had on when I saw her days before. I asked Dad if he could help her change clothes more often, or at least get her to wear her nightgown. But his response was, "do YOU want to try to convince her?"

> **Warning sign: Decreased or poor judgment**
>
> Mom was always a fashionista in her own right. But now, she couldn't make a decision on what to wear, whether it was for a certain occasion, or just based upon the weather. And if we asked her to choose something to wear, she needed a lot of assistance.

A very sad loss

I got the call while on my way to work one morning. Dad had fallen and was in the hospital. That was a wake-up call for us, realizing what a tenuous balance their life was, how one incident could throw everything off kilter. Even though Dad was right across the street in the hospital, there would be no one at home with Mom.

For a week Al and I juggled Mom, Dad, and job, taking turns staying overnight with Mom, arranging for help during the day. Then, sadly, a week after his fall, (on September 4, 2014, one day before their 71st wedding anniversary) we lost Dad, leaving a huge hole in the heart of our family.

Of course we knew that Dad wouldn't be around forever, but there is nothing one can do to prepare for such a loss. Not only was he gone, but we were just starting to realize how much he had been doing for Mom. We continued to take turns staying with Mom, and the more time we spent with her, the more we realized that we had to make a change in her living arrangements.

We considered the possibility of bringing Mom to one of our homes, but the need for 24 hour care made that impossible for either of us. We started to do research on assisted living communities. I really was hoping to have Mom closer to me, of course, and that was my focus. When we found a senior community called Villa St. Benedict, located in Lisle, IL, approximately seven minutes from my home, it seemed to be a good choice.

We really thought that Mom could live in Villa St. Benedict's assisted living community, but it turned out that she needed a lot of extra help. They recommended that we consider moving her to their memory care area, Abbey Lane. At first, we did not agree with that suggestion. It was a process for both Al and me. We were still reeling from the loss of Dad, and if we were to agree to move Mom, we felt we would be losing her as well.

> **Warning sign: Changes in mood and personality**
> Mom would get angry with me, and ask why I always wanted to fight with her. She would call me by one of her sister's names. I would tell her that I was her daughter, not her sister. She would reply with, "since when?" To which I would respond, "Well, since 1948." Then, she would just say, "really?"

We did take our time asking lots of questions, making lots of visits, and in the process, we discovered a calm, nurturing, loving environment. In the end, we saw Mom struggling on her own, so we decided to give Abbey Lane a try. After all, if we couldn't be there "24/7," it was good to know that someone who cared would be with her at all times.

Learning more about Alzheimer's Disease
and Related Dementias (ADRD)

At this point, being confronted head on with Alzheimer's Disease was enough to motivate me to learn even more about it. Up until now, I confess I was still looking for signs that Mom's memory loss was normal for a person her age. Emotionally, that was where I wanted to be. Intellectually, it was not where I was.

It is hard to describe the stress that greets you around every corner. I wanted to know everything that I could about ADRD. Through my experience, I learned that just getting through the day can be daunting. This applies not only to the person affected by it, but to loved ones as well.

It is not like an illness that you can treat. It will not go away. Once it invades, it is here to stay. Because of this, I truly believe it is the most insidious disease of all. The underlying feeling of helplessness never leaves.

Once Mom moved to Villa St. Benedict, I took a closer look at ADRD. I joined the support group there, and was guided to the Alzheimer's Association and their extremely helpful knowledge base. I was able to see more clearly that Mom was exhibiting many of the signs of dementia, not simply old age. I really had not been around anyone who shared this same story. It was such a relief and comfort to be among those who understood, and who could offer support and guidance based on their own personal experiences.

When Dad was caring for Mom, he always would tell us that things were okay. I believe that was *his* way of coping with such a stressful, often heartbreaking, situation. Looking back, I think I probably would have done the same thing. How easy it was for me, looking in from the outside, to judge what he was doing with his beloved wife of almost 71 years.

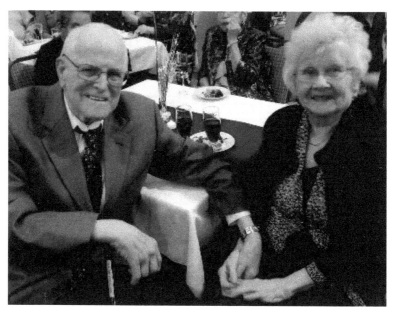

They were known as that couple who always held hands.

2

John, My Dad

They called him St. John. And that was *before* Mom's diagnosis. They (family and friends) knew that he was a man you could always count on. He took care of everything and everyone, it seemed.

But new to us was the term, "caregiver." Dad fell right into that role without us (or him!) even realizing it. Mom and Dad were always together as a team, so it never occurred to us that one was caring more for one than the other. Once we received Mom's diagnosis, I think we just didn't want to believe that it was as serious as it was.

I wanted to know everything I could so that we could "beat it," and right there was my first misconception about ADRD. I really thought it just couldn't be possible that there was no known cure. Surely we could do *something* to make a difference.

Initially I believed we could practice with Mom. We could talk about all of those familiar things in her life, and it would get better. That's how it worked, right? But, she just couldn't do it, no matter how many hints I gave her when I asked her about holidays, seasons, days of the week, family members, etc. So much was lost, and would never return to her memory.

For Dad, the stress of the situation showed up in many ways. Because he was not a man who let on that anything was wrong, I think it was just hard on him, keeping it all to himself. He had health issues of his own, having congestive heart failure. Yet, he soldiered on, taking on much more than he could handle, not wanting to let go. It took its toll.

We weren't looking for signs of caregiver stress, because I'm not sure that we realized the scope of what he was doing for mom. Plus, I still hadn't reconciled the fact that he WAS a caregiver. He was, after all, "Dad." Looking back on those six years, the signs of stress were there. We just didn't know what they were, simply attributing so much to old age. He *was* 87 when they started down this path.

Our concern for him and their safety was validated one day after they had stopped by to visit me. We always asked them to call when they got home, and when a couple of hours passed without a phone call, I called them. There was no answer, and then I started to worry. I called Al, and we decided to wait a little longer. We didn't know if they had already arrived home, and just didn't hear the phone, or were still out on the road somewhere. A scary thought.

About an hour later, they finally answered their phone. Dad said they took a nice tour of Chicago before coming home (which was definitely NOT on their way home!). Apparently, he had made a wrong turn and it took three hours for what would normally be a 45 minute drive. Yet, this was a route they had been taking for about twenty-five years. He acted like it wasn't any big deal. They made it home, didn't they? Yikes!

At that time, my research about Alzheimer's Disease had been all about Mom, but it didn't occur to me to search for information about that other most important person, the caregiver. I would have found out from The Alzheimer's Association about the signs of caregiver stress, and Dad certainly experienced many of them.

- ♦ *"Denial about the disease and its effect on the person who has been diagnosed. "* I believe that Dad just wanted things to be as they had always been, and he would always say "She's okay."

- ♦ *"Anger at the person with Alzheimer's or frustration that he or she can't do the things they used to be able to do."* Actually, it was rare that Dad got angry with Mom. He was not a fighter…rather a peacekeeper. If Mom didn't want to change her clothes, bathe, or eat, he wasn't about to argue with her.

♦ *"Social withdrawal from friends and activities that used to make you feel good."* There were plenty of activities going on at The Devonshire, but Dad did not want to participate in any of them. That should not have been a surprise, since he really didn't participate in much even before they moved there. Mom was the one who was the social butterfly, and pulled him along.

♦ *"Anxiety about the future and facing another day."* I believe that the quickness with which he made the decision to move to the Devonshire was an indication that he didn't know what was going to happen with Mom, especially when she was even more helpless after breaking her wrist.

♦ *"Depression that breaks your spirit and affects your ability to cope."* Sometimes when I visited, Dad would say that he just wanted to jump out the window. He would tear up and say how much he hated being there. In retrospect, I'm not so sure it was the physical place as much as the emotional place he was in.

♦ *"Exhaustion that makes it nearly impossible to complete necessary daily tasks."* He was so spent trying to take care of everything, much of the time when I arrived at their place, both of them would be slumped together, asleep on the sofa.

♦ *"Irritability that leads to moodiness and triggers negative responses and actions."* He was generally courteous and polite, but showed another side of himself when the CNA's tried to come in and help. In no uncertain terms, he chased many of them out of the apartment, saying that they were not needed.

+ **"Lack of concentration** *that makes it difficult to perform familiar tasks."* Al would make plans to pick them up for dinner, and when he would arrive at their apartment, sometimes they were already down in the dining room. We set up reminders for things like doctor appointments and other social events. Sticky notes and sometimes even large pieces of paper were all around the house now.

+ **"Health problems** *that begin to take a mental and physical toll."* Dad focused his energy on Mom's issues, rather than paying a lot of attention to his own health. Congestive heart failure continued to plague him, and even though he wasn't feeling well himself, he would just shuffle along with Mom.

+ **"Sleeplessness** *caused by a never ending list of concerns."* I never observed this, since I wasn't there at night, and of course dad wouldn't mention it, even if it were an issue for him.

Some of these signs were brought to the surface during that wacky trip to New York. We really had planned on dropping down to Virginia to visit my daughter Kiki (their granddaughter). After that harrowing trip just to get to New York, I decided we had to cancel that part of the trip. I was so worried that something would go terribly wrong if we extended it.

Prior to this, I would never have had that thought about my "strong" parents. It was on this trip that I really saw how fragile they both were. I was unwilling to put their lives at risk, by extending our trip.

I know that my dad was terribly disappointed, but the following incident on the way home confirmed that I had made the right decision. When we stopped for the night at the hotel, Dad had to go directly to the bathroom in the hotel lobby. By the time Mom and I checked in, he still had not come out of the bathroom. We knocked on the door and he said that he was okay, but had blood in his urine, and was having a hard time getting himself together.

I immediately asked at the desk where the nearest hospital was. I thought we would be on our way shortly. I then called Al, who said that this had happened before. It had everything to do with Dad's medications. So we decided that I would keep an eye on him, and head home in the morning.

The experience was a revelation of what Dad was going through. Not only was he so concerned about Mom, but, he had his own health issues to deal with. (Such stress!)

Stress relief-what you can do

In our case, there were a couple of ways Dad's stress was relieved. First, Al lived close by, so he had them over for dinner at least once a week, along with another cousin, so there was a good opportunity for some socialization and "getting away." It was a wonderful break for both Dad and Mom, on a regular basis.

We tried to keep things as normal as they ever were. There were a few adjustments. Most holidays they still came to my house or Al's. Or we gathered at the Devonshire for one of their great brunches. Welcome to our "new normal."

Drum therapy

Music was always a part of our lives. Dad was a drummer and a singer in a band, but had retired from that part of his life in his early eighties. He still had his drums, and they made the move with them to The Devonshire, where they sat in the storage area for a while.

One day an entertainer named Joel Palmer came to The Devonshire. He played the guitar and sang lots of the songs that Mom and Dad knew. I was visiting that day, so after the performance, I told him how much we enjoyed it, especially since Dad was a drummer and singer. He then invited Dad to "set up" and play with him the next time he was entertaining.

So, a couple months later, Al and I got those drums out of storage, set up, and then it was the Joel and John show. Residents loved that one of their own was playing, and it elevated Dad to local celebrity status. It improved his mood immensely.

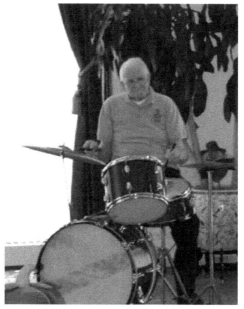

Dad drums at the Devonshire.

Give him a break

When I visited, I tried to do things with Mom to give Dad a little break. We had our "girl" time: shopping, getting her hair done, or going to the knitting/crocheting class. Then, Dad got to be alone for a bit. Many times, though, he would insist on going with us, which was still a "break," by virtue of getting out of the apartment.

If I brought Rufus with me, though, Dad could be convinced to stay home with him. When we returned, it was not unusual for Rufus to have a place of honor on Dad's lap!

Just playing ball and catch with Rufus was a great distraction and lightened his mood. Dad loved it when Rufus came, and in fact he kept a couple of tennis balls and dog dishes in their apartment just for those visits.

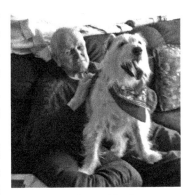

Rufus and Dad

As soon as we arrived, he'd bring out the dishes and fill one with water for Rufus. We would demonstrate the skills that Rufus was learning, and Dad would interact with Rufus to help him hone his skills. He was always amazed at what that crazy little white dog could do.

Animal Assisted Therapy benefits caregivers in many ways. Not only is it a stress reliever, but it can help the caregiver motivate their loved one to accomplish basic daily living tasks.

For instance, eating may be difficult for those with ADRD. When a dog is present a person may be motivated to eat by feeding the dog from a fork, then feeding themselves. (using two different utensils, of course!). If there is a reluctance about getting dressed, the caregiver may want to talk about getting the dog "dressed," then the person. Or the dog can "assist" by bringing articles of clothing to the person (socks, shoes, etc.). Rufus was happy to pick up a sock or shoe and bring it to Mom or Dad. He did expect a treat in return!

Although they lived in a fairly large community, with pleasant walking areas and paths, Mom and Dad rarely took advantage of them. There was a lovely lake with a path around it, with benches strategically located so residents could stop and rest. On many occasions I tried to get them to take a walk with me, but was seldom successful. However, on days that Rufus visited, they would happily take him for a walk with me, and they often suggested that I just leave him with them.

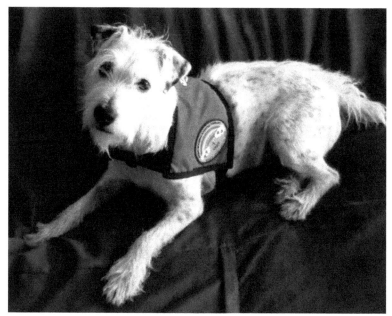

Rufus is proud of the work he does.

connections

PART II

Animal Assisted Therapy

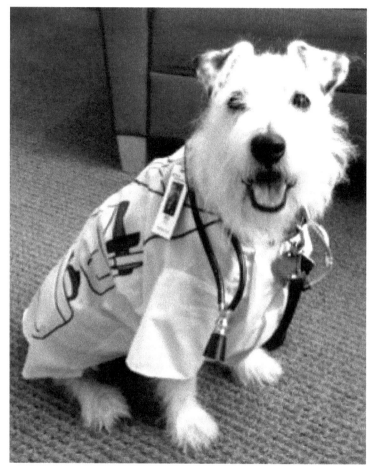

"Dr. Dog"

3

Rufus, Therapy Dog

I learned about Animal Assisted Therapy shortly before we welcomed a cute little Jack Russell Terrier named Rufus into our lives. Would this lively little guy make a good therapy dog?

Our goal with this new little ball of fur was for him to become part of our family. We were lucky to find a "personal trainer" who would come to our home, and show us all how to get along harmoniously.

Generally, dogs need to be at least one year old before beginning therapy dog classes, so when Rufus was a year old, I started my research. I was very lucky to find a group named Rainbow Animal Assisted Therapy, headquartered in Morton Grove, IL, and we never looked back. Most recently, Rufus earned another registration with Alliance of Therapy Dogs, which enables him to broaden his repertoire.

If you know anything about Jack Russell Terriers, you understand why it took a couple of tries to pass his first test with Rainbow Animal Assisted Therapy. In order to pass the final test, teams need to pass every part of it. It is 100% or nothing!

I was so proud of Rufus right up until the very last part, which was to "sit still while petting." When the examiner finally got around to Rufus, he couldn't contain his joy, and with tail wagging furiously, he just about leaped up into the examiner's arms. FAIL.

Another thing about Jack Russell Terriers (and maybe their owners, too!) is that they are very persistent and focused. So, we turned right around and signed up for another class. After all, we both still had a LOT to learn about the therapy dog business.

That was ten years ago, and Rufus is still working his magic with people of all ages. Over the years we've worked in schools, hospitals, libraries and other organizations who request therapy dogs through Rainbow. We have taught dog safety classes. We have a variety of experiences under our belt (or collar, in Rufus's case!).

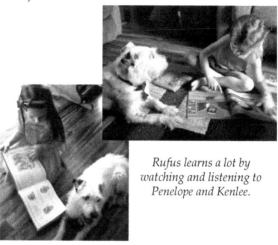

Rufus learns a lot by watching and listening to Penelope and Kenlee.

Living with a therapy dog has its advantages. I discovered that dogs just seem to know when they are needed, and over the years, Rufus has been a bright spot with our family and friends.

When we visit hospitals, he will seek out the patient, and sit quietly near them, most often on their feet. People who meet him while we are "working" say, "I can't believe he's a Jack Russell Terrier, he's so calm." Then, people who visit us at home say, "I can't believe he's a therapy dog, he's so crazy."

Make no mistake. True to his breed, Rufus is one smart dog. When Mom was sent to rehab after that hospital stay, I took him to visit her, "off the clock." Without his signature therapy vest, he was just our family dog. When he saw Mom, he leaped right up onto her bed, something he would never do when we are working.

Through our work as a therapy team, we have had the good fortune to have met so many great people (young and old) over the years. Rufus has worked his magic with young patients at Central DuPage Hospital's pediatric unit, has listened intently to children reading to him at the Wheaton Library, and has comforted patients at Good Samaritan Hospital's oncology and palliative care units.

But, most of all, I knew that my parents always loved it when Rufus visited their home. His importance to them was even more apparent after Mom was diagnosed with ADRD. Mom would always be happy to see him, and a connection was always made. It wasn't uncommon for me to turn around and see Rufus sitting in her lap, or next to her on the sofa.

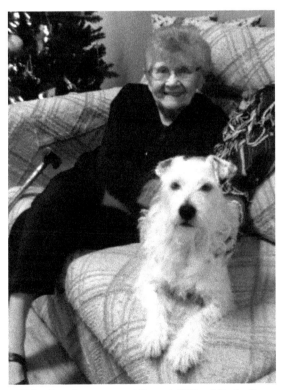

Who doesn't want to pet the cute little white dog?

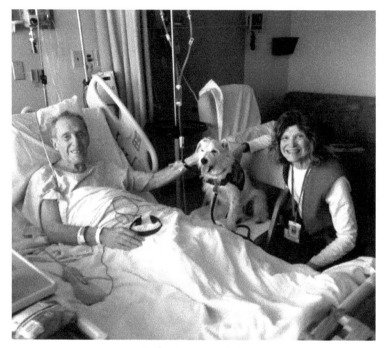

Rufus is good medicine.

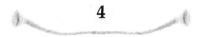

4

Dogs as Therapy

Without exception, Rufus could energize Mom, bring a smile to her face, or help to initiate conversation. This did not come as a surprise to me and Rufus, since we saw small miracles every time we visited a school, hospital, library, or any other facility. However, visiting those with ADRD was very different from what we had experienced so far. Yet the principles remained the same. A life is enriched, a connection is made by the presence of the animal.

I got to spend time with Mom at Villa St. Benedict almost every day of the week and often brought Rufus with me because Mom just loved him. Sometimes we would go back to my home, and there she would enjoy visiting with him.

No matter where, he could always put a smile on her face. When Rufus licked her nose, it was almost pure joy for her, with a tiny bit of "yuck." It was just short of miraculous. Rufus had been in her life for twelve years, and she always loved seeing him, right from that very first Christmas Day when we brought that wiggly little white puppy over to her home to meet her and the rest of the family.

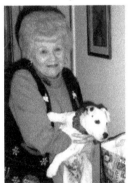

Love at first sight.

Rufus was always a welcome guest at Villa St. Benedict. We soon discovered that not only Mom enjoyed his visits, but other residents were delighted to see him as well. Our experiences had already shown the extraordinary benefits of Animal Assisted Therapy in a variety of settings, and this was no exception.

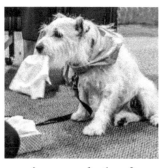

Anyone need a tissue?

It is not just the participant who benefits from the animal's visits, it's the staff, the caregivers, the family and friends. It is all of those people who are part of that person's life. In the hospital, nurses and doctors and other staff get a "shot in the arm" when they see Rufus, especially when he does his signature move, handing a tissue to anyone who sneezes.

His reputation precedes him at Good Samaritan Hospital and we get asked all the time, "is that the dog who gives you a tissue?" The staff always takes time to give him a pat, and he takes the time to give them a paw or a high five. Many of the hospital staff even keep treats in their drawers for those lucky therapy dogs who get to visit.

Functional fitness and making a connection

Animal Assisted Therapy activities for those with ADRD are focused on a combination of two things: making a connection, and *maintaining* functional fitness.

Functional fitness in the athletic world refers to the ability to run, jump, throw, catch, kick, etc. By the time we reach the latter stages of life, functional fitness is about maintaining the ability to walk, get up and down a flight of stairs, get in and out of a car, brush your teeth, your hair, eat with utensils, mentally connect the dots, and much more. As we grow older, our athletic abilities and mental functions naturally tend to deteriorate.

It is at these latter stages where Animal Assisted Therapy can be helpful. Why? Because unlike a fellow human, a dog is non-judgmental and non-threatening. People will do things with and for a dog that they will not otherwise do. Animal Assisted Therapy for those with dementia is all about *maintaining* function. "Use it or lose it."

All the functions of daily living are so important in order to maintain independence. It's not how you look, but what you can do. The activities in this book will help people with ADRD *maintain* functional fitness, mentally and/or physically.

The facilitator and goal directed therapy

As good as Rufus is, he still needs a bit of human input to work his magic. We are a team. The dog is the motivator and the human is the facilitator who makes the therapy work.

For example, when working with a participant who needs assistance with a cognitive skill such as language, there are any number of activities that can be of value. The simplest would be for the participant to give a verbal command. The facilitator would make sure that the dog is not only in the proper position to receive the command, but has its focus on the participant.

Or, if a participant needs assistance with an everyday skill such as eating, the participant can hold a utensil, put food on the utensil, and feed the dog. The facilitator may provide guidance so that the participant can be successful at the task.

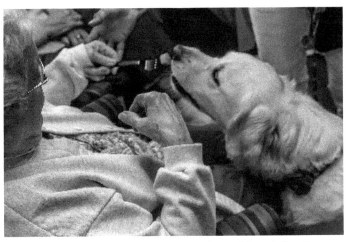

The handler facilitates by guiding the participant's hand

The facilitator guides the participant by letting him/her know when to give the command. Once the command is obeyed, the facilitator makes sure that the dog is given its expected reward. Most often this is a treat, although some dogs respond to a scratch behind the ears. Rufus is not one of those dogs!

Every time a visit is made, it is critical to have a plan for what is to be accomplished during that visit (Goal Directed Therapy). It can be as uncomplicated as a session of reaching out and petting the dog, or as involved as implementing a game, such as the dice game (Described on page 64), that uses multiple skills.

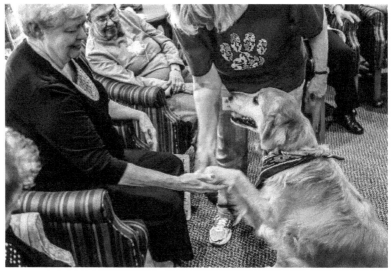

Zoe gets a little help

The effects of Animal Assisted Therapy

Research shows that Animal Assisted Therapy is effective in so many ways because it lowers levels of cortisol, our "fight or flight" hormone. It also increases levels of serotonin our "feel good" hormone. All of this means that the interaction can help to lower heart rates, blood pressure, stress levels, cholesterol levels, and could even protect against heart disease. The increased physical activity that is encouraged by the animal is a large contributor to these benefits.

The benefits of the interaction can be broadly categorized into three areas: Cognitive, Social and Physical. In most cases, Animal Assisted Therapy activities reap multiple benefits.

As it relates to ADRD, the therapy activities described in this book focus on *maintaining* functional fitness and making connections through specific aspects of these three categories. Some of the benefits are described below:

Cognitive, Psychological, Emotional
+ Lower stress
+ Decrease depression
+ Reduce agitation, verbally disruptive behaviors
+ Increase focus and attention on a task

Physical,. Motor
+ Improve fine motor skills
+ Improve hand-eye coordination
+ Improve gait skills, wheelchair mobility
+ Improve range of motion
+ Increase functional fitness; sitting, standing, etc.
+ Increase strength to improve daily living activities
+ Decrease in pain, even a possible decrease in medications

Social, Daily Living)
+ Enhance communication about feelings
+ Enhance social behavior in small groups

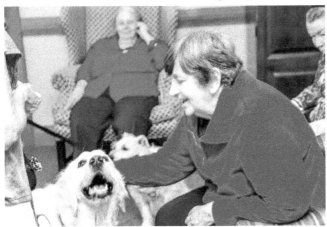

Rufus and Izzy's visit reaps many benefits

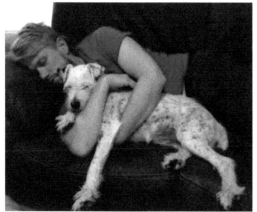

*Our Family Dogs
are always
there for us*

*Rufus excels at cuddling and napping,
especially with Cody.*

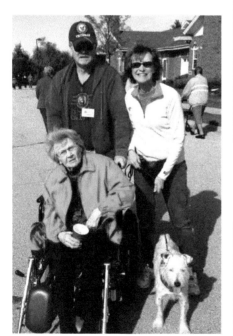

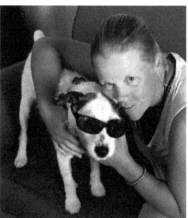

Rock star Rocket and Kiki

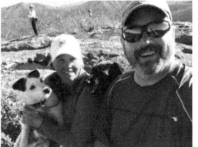

*At the Alzheimer's Walk
Mom, Al, Rufus and me.*

*Rocket and Scherzer enjoy
a hike with Kiki and Adam.*

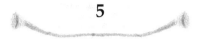

5

Family Pets as Therapy

If you don't have access to a therapy team, and if you are looking for a way to make a connection with someone in your care or someone you know who has ADRD, consider the fact that your family dog can be your own personal therapy dog. Research shows that when a person with ADRD has a pet, they are inclined to demonstrate more interactive behavior; sometimes aimed at the dog more than at another person. But a connection is made, nonetheless.

Many of the activities don't require a lot of extra training other than basic obedience and a dog who is already a good family member. Even simple commands such as "sit", "come," and "stay" are valuable in encouraging language and making a connection. Here are some activities with which your own pet can help in making a connection. More details can be found on the pages indicated next to each activity:

Sitting on Lap, or next to, Petting (page 50)
Feeding (page 55)
Read Book Aloud (page 67)
Brush Dog (page 76)
Dressing (page 81)
Style Hair (page 96)
Walk the Dog (page 122)

As an example, common simple commands can be turned into a game. You can make cards with the commands printed on them, and play "pick a card." Depending on cognitive level, the participant can read the card, then give the dog the command (Explained later under Cards and Skills, page 62).

More suggestions are found in Chapter 10. Simple commands that most family dogs respond to (such as Shake, High five, Sit up, Down, Crawl, Roll over) have therapy value because any interaction with the dog encourages a connection, starting with language (giving the command).

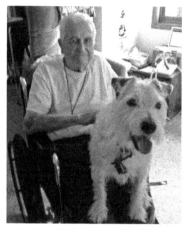

Start by making a list of skills your dog already is able to do. It might be surprising how many your dog already possesses. Does your dog love to jump up on the sofa and curl up next to you, or sit in your lap? Does your dog sit quietly next to you or on your feet? For someone with ADRD, who may be frustrated, confused or anxious, a warm calm furry dog may be just what is needed.

Rufus calmly warms Glen's lap.

Or, if you're looking for some physical activity, focused on functional fitness, does your dog drop a ball or toy at your feet, looking expectantly at you? Your loved one can take it from him, or pick it up and play a game of catch. How about going for a walk? Mobility is a big part of keeping functionally fit, and taking a walk is just the start. It involves other cognitive functions such as concentration, focus on the dog, language. motor planning and sequencing.

Think about some other functional daily living skills, such as putting on clothing. Does your dog have a sweater he wears that a person can put on for him? Or, have some fun with sunglasses or hats.

So many possibilities begin with a simple connection. All those animal behaviors we so enjoy and take for granted can be incorporated into meaningful and therapeutic interventions for your family member with ADRD.

Nasha. Lap dog.

6

Individualizing Animal Assisted Therapy Activities to Participants' Cognitive levels

In order to maximize the benefits of Animal Assisted Therapy with those affected by ADRD, it is important to understand that there is a wide range of cognitive abilities among the individual participants. If you have never had experience or been in contact with a person affected by ADRD, it can be intimidating or confusing. It is a "normal" to which many have not been exposed

Modify

Each of the following activities can be modified to a participant's cognitive/functional level. There are criteria outlined by the National Institute on Aging, the Alzheimer's Association, and many other related organizations that can help you tailor interactions with participants at an appropriate cognitive/functional level.

The criteria used for categorizing activities in this book correspond to some commonly used assessment tools by health professionals:

- The Reisberg Scale (Global Deterioration Scale for Assessment of Primary Degenerative Dementia (GDS) focuses on cognition.
- The Reisberg Functional Assessment Staging (FAST) Scale focuses on a person's functional level as it relates to daily living activities.
- The Clinical Dementia Rating (CDR) Scale focuses on a combination of both cognition and function.
- The Allen Cognitive Assessment Battery also takes into consideration both cognition and function.

A User Friendly Guide

To create a user friendly guide for AAT teams, family members, health professionals and other users of this book, the suitable cognitive/functional impairment level is indicated throughout and appears at the beginning of each activity:

Suitable Cognitive/Functional Impairment Level

Mild	Moderate	Severe

This activity would correspond to FAST scale, stages 1-4:
Ranging from no memory difficulties to increased forgetfulness, difficulty concentrating, memory decrease, social withdrawal, difficulty managing everyday tasks, decreased job functionality, difficulty traveling to new locations.

Suitable Cognitive/Functional Impairment Level

Mild	Moderate	Severe

This activity would correspond to FAST scale, stages 5-6 characterized by, in addition to the above:
Decreased ability to dress, bathe, toilet, requiring assistance with these tasks.
Loss of sense of time or place, little memory of recent events. In addition, urinary or fecal incontinence.

Suitable Cognitive/Functional Impairment Level

Mild	Moderate	Severe

This activity would correspond to FAST scale, stage 7 characterized by, in addition to the above:
Loss of speech, motor skills, possibly consciousness.
Limited verbal ability. A few words per day.
Intelligible vocabulary lost.
Unable to walk, smile, even hold up head.

Suggestions and methods are provided to adapt an activity as needed to accommodate various levels. If the participant does not understand or is unable to perform the activity, then it usually can be modified.

Remember, these are simply guidelines. The more you work with people who have ADRD, the more you will be accustomed to using your good judgement about what can or cannot be accomplished.

Have patience

Working with those who have ADRD requires patience, the ability to slow down, direct eye contact, listening closely, and responding appropriately. Interacting with a person who for the most part lives in the moment is a challenge, and requires a calm, accepting demeanor all of which a therapy dog offers.

Here are some general guidelines I've found helpful:
- Introduce yourself and your dog each and every visit.
- Speak loudly
- Speak slowly.
- Speak clearly.
- Repeat as many times as needed.
- Look directly at participant when speaking.
- Break down the activity one step at a time. The participant may not be able to "sequence."
- Always give instructions in the same way. Simple, without using lots of other words, which could lead to confusion.
- Show participants HOW to give the treat to the dog, with open palm. Explain every time, if needed.
- Be aware of participants' fragility, especially when the dog is reaching out to them. A hard claw may tear fragile, delicate thin skin.
- Demonstrate and assist.
- Be patient.
- Pace the number of planned activities. Don't overload.

Keep in mind that in addition to cognitive challenges, people with ADRD are often visually or hearing impaired. Depth perception, and field of vision may be affected, and a participant may have difficulty seeing objects. Sometimes a participant sees me, but not Rufus, because he's not in the field of vision. I then lift him up and say that Rufus is here, too, which generally prompts a smile, some conversation, and a hand reaching out to touch him.

Items used in activities such as the ball, dice, hoop, etc. are sometimes not seen by a participant. After explaining an activity, it is important to be close to the participant not only to place an object in a hand, but for the dog to be positioned within sight or touch.

Always interact with dignity and respect. As a family member, I so appreciated the many people who spent time with my mom, and treated her as a healthy person. Above all, listen. You never know what you'll learn from folks with so many interesting life experiences.

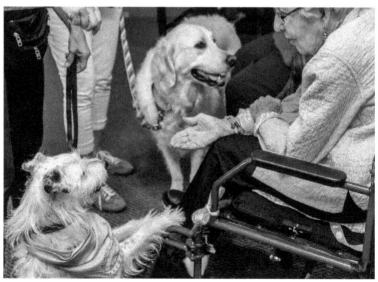

Rufus and Izzy respectfully greet new friends.

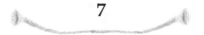

7

What's in your bag?
Suggested equipment

Rufus and I have certain standard pieces of equipment that are always in a bag and ready to go. A box of tissues is a must for his "signature move." An extra leash, water bowl, plastic cups, hoop, blindfold, book, dice and skill list, bandana for a blindfold, and a puzzle are our staples.

Here is a list of items I usually have on hand, and move in and out of my therapy equipment bags. It depends on where Rufus and I are heading, the people with whom we are working, and their cognitive/functional level.

Add your own creative ideas!

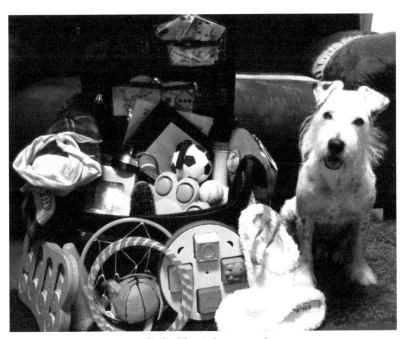

Rufus likes to be prepared.

Suggested items for your bag:

+ Extra leash
+ Water bowl and water
+ Large rubber dice
+ Laminated page or two of skills your dog can do, numbered from 2-12 (for dice, spinner game)
+ Customized picture cards with name of skills on them
+ Simple books, newspapers and magazines for participants to read aloud to dog
+ Plastic buckets (usually from ice cream gallons)
+ Soft "bean bags" made from socks and foam rubber
+ Sturdy plastic or small metal fork for feeding
+ Barrettes, clips for "styling" dog's hair
+ Bandanas, scarves, to "dress" the dog
+ Soft slippers for dog to bring to participant
+ Plastic cups of various colors
+ Soft balls, various sizes, types
+ Bowling ball and pins
+ Box of tissues
+ Sports cone(s)
+ Doggie bubbles
+ Bell(s)
+ Tambourine
+ Dog puzzle
+ Children's piano
+ Tunnel
+ Hoop
+ Basketball Hoop
+ Buzzers
+ Brush

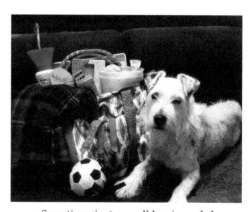

Sometimes just a small bag is needed.

connections

PART III

Animal Assisted Therapy Activities

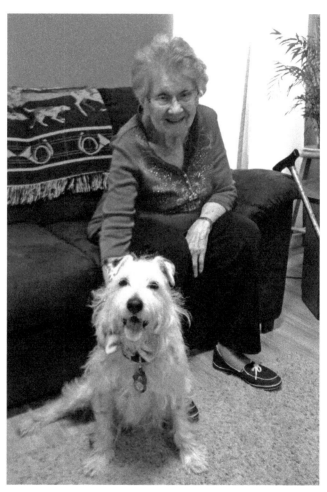

So happy together

8

Irene's Favorites

There were many activities that Mom liked to do with Rufus, but her favorite was just having him close to her so that she could pet and talk to him. She really liked to give him commands. I think it gave her a sense of empowerment, when her life at this stage afforded very little opportunity for her to "take charge." With Rufus as a willing participant, they were quite a team.

Rufus knew that if he brought the ball to Mom and placed it in her hand, she would "get in the game." When food was around, he was first in line to offer assistance! When Mom was faced with physical therapy prescribed to improve her strength and functional fitness, Rufus encouraged and motivated her in a way that I or the therapist could not. Following are some of Mom's favorite activities with Rufus.

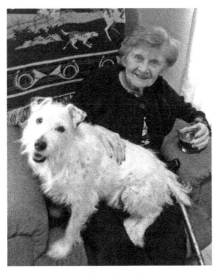

A match made in heaven

🐾🐾 Sitting on Lap, or Next to, Petting.

Suitable Cognitive/Functional Impairment Level

Mild	Moderate	Severe

Connection:

Cognitive: Language, attention

Motor: Range of motion, hand-eye coordination, Manual dexterity

Social: Caring for others, Expressing feelings, Meeting, Greeting, Starting conversations, Staying calm

Procedure:

Ask participant if it's okay for the dog to sit next to them. Or if it's a small dog, in their lap or next to them on a sofa, etc.

Modification: Handler could sit near participant with dog on lap, accessible to participant.

Tip: If you're working with a participant with severe cognitive impairment, be sure to have a caregiver let you know how the participant feels about dogs. Will they enjoy the close contact, touch of a dog? Is it okay to place the dog next to them or on a lap? Communicate to the participant what you are going to do. NO surprises.

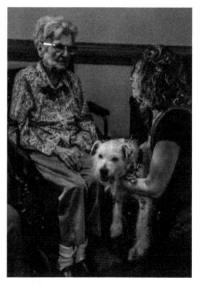

Rufus says hello from a distance.

No matter where my mom sat, Rufus would end up in her lap, or at least next to her. Of course, that could have had something to do with the distinct possibility that he would be fed some delectable morsel from her.

Never underestimate the power of the mere presence of a dog in the life of a person with ADRD. The simple touch of a dog can prompt a smile, or inspire mobility. Almost always the dog conjures up a nurturing caring attitude that seems to stir memories and stimulate conversation, such as, "My dog used to..."

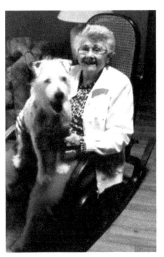

Let's rock!

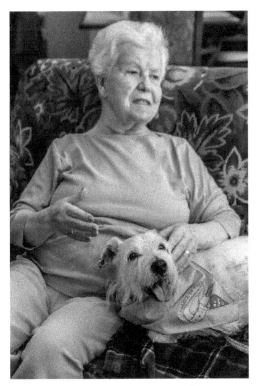

Rufus encourages conversation.

51

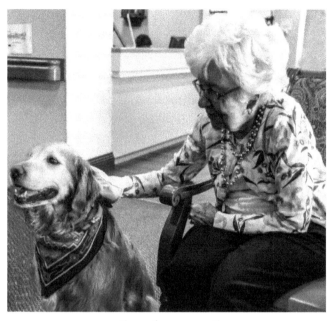

Zoe makes a connection.

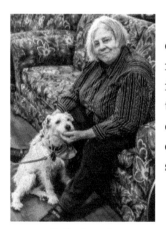

Rufus leans in.

Residents at Abbey Lane just enjoy having Rufus next to them, or reaching down to pat him. Since Rufus is a small dog, when he sits or lies next to them, I tell them that they'll have to reach down to pet him because he's short. One of the residents told me, "that's okay, I'm short, too!"

Sometimes all it takes is a gentle touch to make someone's day. Brightie has that magic touch, as she waits patiently to greet a participant.

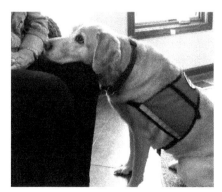

Gentle Brightie

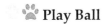 Play Ball

Suitable Cognitive/Functional Impairment Level

Mild	Moderate	Severe

Mom loved to play ball with Rufus. She would even try to "trick" Rufus by pretending to throw, then releasing it so he could chase the ball. Or she would play catch with him, by tossing the ball in the air, so he could catch it.

Connection:
Cognitive: Language, Reasoning, Sequencing
Motor: Grasp objects, Hand-eye coordination, Manual dexterity, Range of motion,
Social: Teamwork, Control

Equipment:
Ball (soft nerf type, tennis ball)

Procedure:
Participant holds ball.
Participant throws ball.
Dog retrieves ball, puts it in participant's hand.

Tip: Use a very soft ball, in case of errant throws. Participant and/or handler can count the number of throws.

Modification:
Participant can play catch with the dog, instead of the dog chasing the ball. Participant throws the ball to the dog, who catches it, and then places ball in participant's hand.

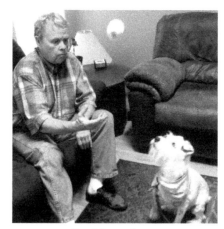

Participant throws.

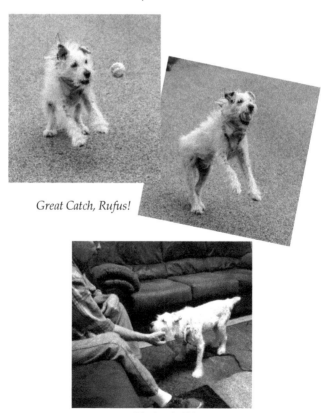

Great Catch, Rufus!

*Placing ball in
Participant's hand.*

Feeding

Suitable Cognitive/Functional Impairment Level

Mild	Moderate	Severe

Connection:
Cognitive: Follow directions, Language, Perception, Sequencing, Visual and Spatial processing
Motor: Grasp objects, Manual dexterity, Range of motion
Social: Asking questions, Caring for others, Cooperation, Eye contact, Feeding, Sharing

Equipment:
Sturdy plastic fork or small metal fork
Bowl with lid to hold suitable snacks that can be speared with the fork (We generally use cooked carrot slices, cauliflower, broccoli, or even small cheese chunks)

Procedure:
Position dog in front of or next to participant.
Give participant a fork or spoon, and a container with the food.
Participant puts food on fork or spoon.
Participant feeds dog with utensil.

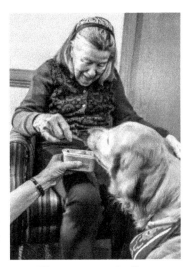

Modification:
Handler can hold container with food for the dog, allowing the participant to simply "spear" the food, and feed. Food can be placed in open hand without utensil.

Have more carrots, Zoe.

Mom was always asking if Rufus had eaten, because she wanted to feed him. Rufus loved to sit near her because he knew that she would always be good for a bite or two. She was great for feeding him from the table, or from wherever she was sitting.

In the case of a person with ADRD, this activity should be monitored very closely, since that person may not understand or remember that certain foods are not good for dogs. In Mom's case, it was a continuous battle with the chocolate she loved, which is toxic to dogs. She couldn't resist Rufus's wide eyes that said "it's really okay to feed me chocolate."

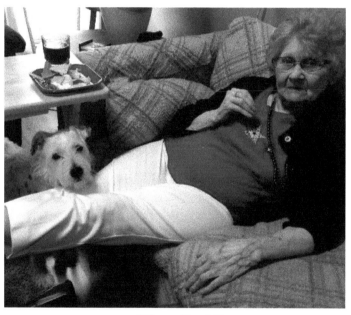

Who could resist?

Eating is an issue with many who are affected by ADRD. They may not remember what, or even if, they ate. Or that they are eating while they are sitting at a table. Feeding Rufus was one of Mom's favorites, and is something that can be motivating, when a person takes turns feeding the dog with a fork, then eating a bite themselves. This is a great activity to promote a connection with the caregiver and the participant.

Tip: Keep a close eye to be sure that the participant doesn't eat from the fork that is intended for the dog, or feed the dog food that is not good for dogs.

This activity is also a great conversation starter. It encourages questions about what dogs eat in general, and sometimes on a personal level of what their own dogs used to eat. The participants never cease to be amazed that the dogs actually like the different foods they feed them from a fork, such as carrots and cauliflower. The conversation can go in several directions, such as what foods are good to eat, etc. Research has shown that many people will eat more after the dog visits.

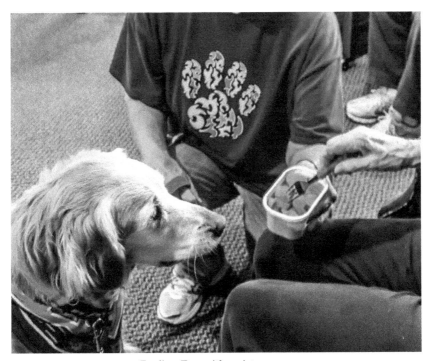

Feeding Zoe, with assistance

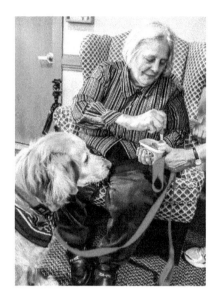

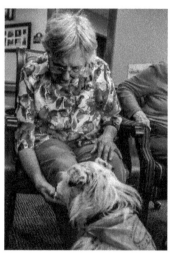

Zoe (top) and Izzy (bottom) prefer to eat daintily from a fork, while Rufus prefers a more slobbery, direct route by hand!

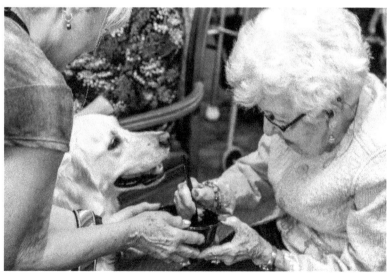

🐾 Sitting and standing

Suitable Cognitive/Functional Impairment Level

Mild	Moderate	Severe

When Mom was given certain exercises to assist with her functional fitness, Rufus was there to lend a hand. One of her "exercises" was simply to transition from sitting to standing. This can be a challenge, and sometimes difficult to remember for someone with ADRD.

By watching Rufus stand, then sit, then stand, then sit, Mom would do her required amount of "reps" with ease. Sometimes she would count out loud how many times she would sit and stand, which encouraged language.

Connection:
Cognitive: Follow directions, Language, Memory, Numbers, Sequencing
Motor: Balance, Mobility, Range of motion
Social: Cooperation, Eye contact

Equipment:
Chair

Procedure:
Participant sits in chair.
Dog sits, facing participant.
Participant stands.
Dog stands as participant stands.
Participant sits.
Dog sits as participant sits.
Repeat!

Modification:
Participant can give verbal commands to dog to sit or stand.

> **Tip**: Handler can give dog a hand signal to sit and stand, so it appears that the dog is responding to the visual and verbal stimulus of the participant.

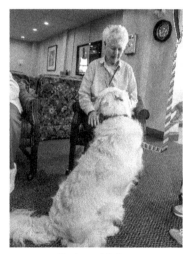

Sitting with Izzy

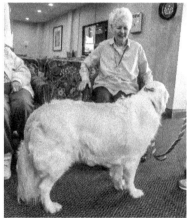

Izzy offers encouragement to stand.

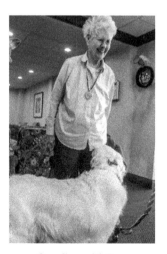

Standing with Izzy

9

Cognitive, Psychological, Emotional Connections

By engaging in the activities in this chapter, cognitive, psychological and emotional connections are encouraged. While this is the main focus, social and motor skills are involved as well. Whether the participant is giving a command or simply communicating with the dog during an activity, language is encouraged. Movement plays a role as the participant sorts, grasps, or tosses the objects involved in a specific activity or game. So many skills which may have diminished over time in a participant are reinforced while participating and interacting with the dog. In the end, the overall goal is to spark a connection.

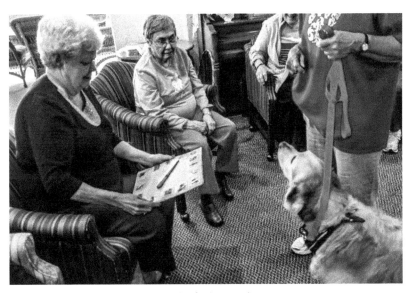

Zoe waits for instructions.

🐾 Card and skill Game

Suitable Cognitive/Functional Impairment Level

Mild	Moderate	Severe

Connection:
Cognitive: Communication, Decision making, Language, Numbers, Reading, Reasoning
Motor: Grasp objects, Hand-eye coordination, Manual dexterity, Range of motion
Social: Control, Cooperation, Eye contact, Teamwork

Equipment:
Cards with photo and text of dog's skills on them
Equipment pictured on the skill cards:
Tunnel
Brush
Cups
Fork and food to feed dog
Tissue
Hoop
Puzzle

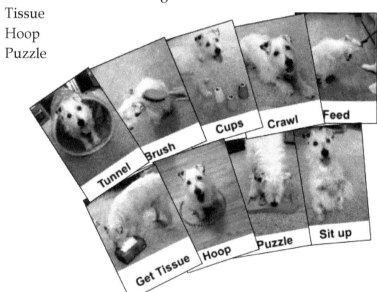

Procedure:
Participant is seated, with dog next to him/her.
Handler holds out cards to participant, face down.
Participant picks card.
Participant reads the skill.
Participant gives dog the verbal command.
Participant gives dog a treat.

Modification:
Handler can assist with reading the card and giving command.
Participant can give the treat, with assistance.

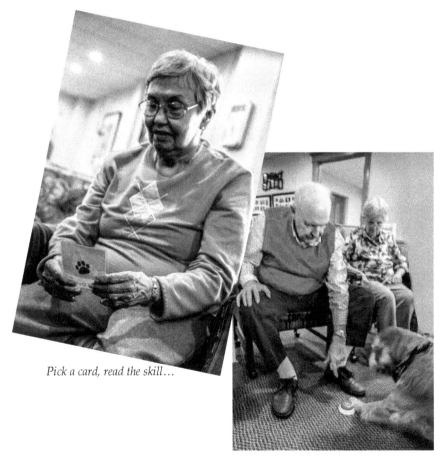

Pick a card, read the skill…

…and the card says "buzzer."

🐾 Dice and skill Game

Suitable Cognitive/Functional Impairment Level

Mild	Moderate	Severe

Connection:
Cognitive: Attention, Language, Numbers, Reading, Sequencing
Motor: Grasping objects, Manual dexterity, Range of motion
Social: Control, Eye contact, Sharing, Teamwork

Equipment:
Large, soft dice
Skill list, numbered from 2-12, preferably with picture of skill next to the number, and name of skill
Other equipment as needed for each skill. i.e., hoop, cups, etc.

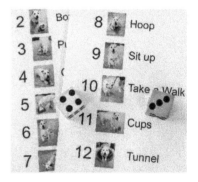

Procedure:
Participant is seated, with dog next to him/her.
Hand dice to participant.
Participant is instructed to "throw" dice on the ground.
Participant counts the number of dots on the dice.
Dog brings the dice back to participant.
Participant finds the corresponding number on the chart
Dog is given the verbal command for the skill.

Tip: The game can be played with a group. Cooperation is encouraged by involving several participants. One can throw the dice, another can count, another can read the skill and another can have the dog perform the skill.

Modification

Handler can lend more assistance by counting the dots on the dice, or reading the skill, if participant is unable to do so.

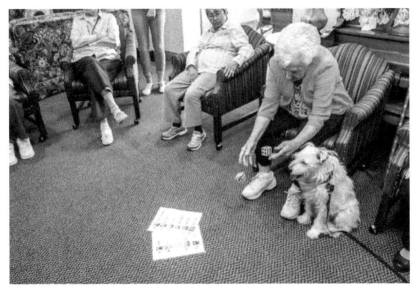

Rufus waits for the "throw."

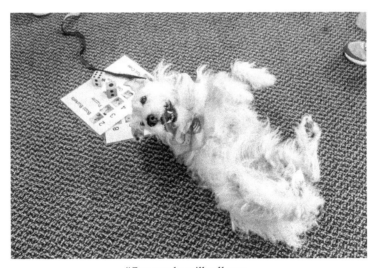

#7 means he will roll over.

Hoop

Suitable Cognitive/Functional Impairment Level

Mild	Moderate	Severe

Connection:
Cognitive: Language, Attention, Visual and spatial processing
Motor: Grasp objects, Hand-eye coordination, Manual dexterity
Social: Control, Cooperation, Interaction with dog

Equipment:
Hoop

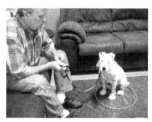

Procedure:
Handler places hoop on the floor.
Participant gives command "go in."
Dog walks to hoop and sits within it.

Rufus goes "in."

Participant gives command to "come out."
Dog walks to participant.
Participant can hold hoop and tell dog to "go through," "over," or "under."

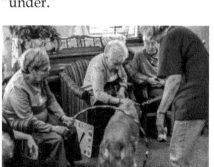

Tip: Concepts such as "in," "out," "through,", "over," "under." are reinforced.

Modification: Handler can hold hoop with participant, and dog can jump through.

Zoe goes "through."

🐾🐾 Read book aloud
(or newspaper, magazine, etc.)

Suitable Cognitive/Functional Impairment Level

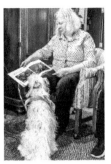

Rufus gets a closer look.

Mild	Moderate	Severe

Connection:

Cognitive: Language, Reading (a skill that is often diminished with ADRD)

Motor: Grasp objects, Manual dexterity

Social: Cooperation, Expressing feelings, Initiate conversation, Listening skills, Teamwork

Equipment:
Books, magazines, newspapers

Tip: Choose easy to read materials, depending upon your participants. Children's books would work well, and the participant could be told that the book is a favorite of the dog. (Rufus actually has his own book, entitled "Rufus T. Dog." I tell participants that this is his favorite book because it's all about him.)

Procedure:
Position dog sitting next to participant, either on a sofa, or the dog can sit at participant's feet.
Handler hands the book to participant.
Participant reads the book out loud to the dog.

Modification:
This is also a good group activity. The book can be passed around the room, so each person can read one page while others listen.

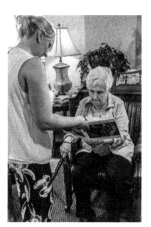

Handler can read book out loud if participant is unable to do so.
Reading magazines or newspapers will also stimulate conversation.

Staff help facilitate.

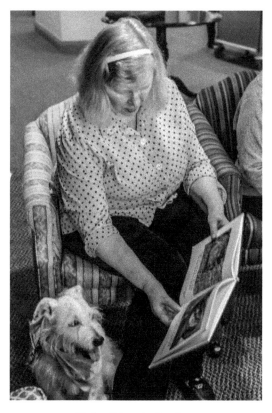

Rufus listens to the story.

🐾 Sort Objects by Color-Bucket Game

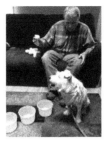

Suitable Cognitive/Functional Impairment Level

Mild	Moderate	Severe

Let the game begin.

Connection:
Cognitive: Colors, Follow directions, Language, Memory, Perception, Sorting, Visual and spatial processing
Motor: Grasp objects, Hand-eye coordination, Manual dexterity, Range of motion, Upper body movement
Social: Control, Cooperation, Initiate conversations, Interaction with dog

Equipment:
Small to medium plastic buckets
Beanbags, rolled up socks, other lightweight objects to "toss"
Other objects of various colors suitable for sorting

Procedure:
Handler sets three small plastic "buckets" in a row in front of the participant.
Participant is shown the "beanbags" and is asked to sort, or choose "like" colors.
Participant then puts (or tosses) the socks into buckets.
Dog will retrieve them from the buckets, give back to participant.
If the participant misses a bucket, dog will retrieve it, and give it back to participant for another try.
Then, move to the next person.

Modification:
Objects of different colors can be sorted, (i.e., balls, beanbags, etc.) and the buckets can be used to keep them organized as the participant sorts the items.

> Tip: This is also a great individual activity that caregivers can enjoy with the participant. In addition, the dog can take a turn by being given one of the objects to "put in" a bucket. Score can be kept, tracking how many beanbags the participant successfully throws in the buckets vs. how many the dog drops in.

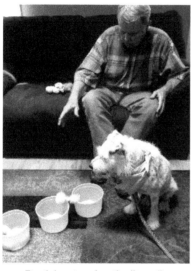

Participant makes the "toss."

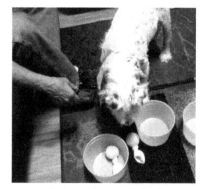

Rufus retrieves a "miss."

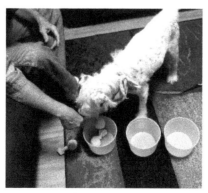

It's Rufus's turn to put it in.

🐾 Sort Objects by Shape

Suitable Cognitive/Functional Impairment Level

Mild	Moderate	Severe

Connection:
Cognitive: Attention, Memory, Perception, Sorting (shapes), Sequencing, Visual and spatial processing
Motor: Grasp objects, Hand-eye coordination, Manual dexterity
Social: Cooperation, Interaction with dog

Equipment:
Various shaped objects
Corresponding shape game

Procedure:
Explain how to hide the treats in the game.
Show participant a variety of shapes.
Ask participant to pick out the shape that can be used to hide the treats.
Dog is blindfolded.
Participant places treat in the game.
Participant places shape into corresponding spot.
Participant asks dog to "find it."

Modification:
To simplify, you can use a puzzle that has all of the same shapes. In this case the round and square shapes can be sorted first, in order to determine which shapes go with which puzzle. Once that is determined, the activity can proceed.

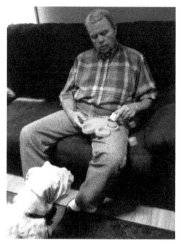

*Placing circle shapes.
Rufus is blindfolded.*

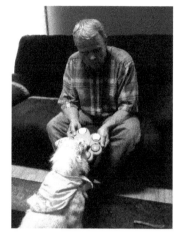

Rufus ponders his options.

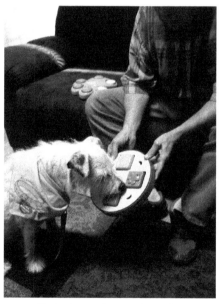

*Rufus hopes the treat is under
the red square.*

🐾 Spinner and skill Game

Suitable Cognitive/Functional Impairment Level

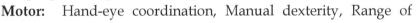

Mild	Moderate	Severe

Connection:
Cognitive: Follow directions, Language, Perception, Reading
Motor: Hand-eye coordination, Manual dexterity, Range of motion
Social: Control, Cooperation, Eye contact, Initiate conversations, Teamwork

Equipment:
Spinner (can be customized, or contain numbers or colors that correspond to skills on your list)
Equipment designated on the spinner (tunnel, puzzle, etc.)

Procedure:
Participant is seated, with dog next to him/her.
Handler holds out spinner and instructs participant to "spin it."
Participant reads corresponding skill pointed out by the spinner.
Participant gives dog the designated verbal command.

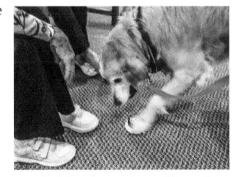

> Tip: For a larger group, one person can spin, one can read the skill, and still another can give the command

And the spinner points to "Buzzer."

Modification:
Handler can spin for the participant.

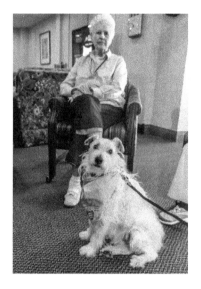

Ready, set…

Connect!!

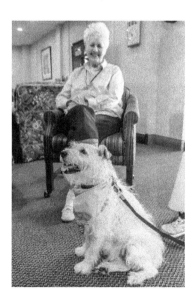

10

Social, Daily Living Connections

The focus of this chapter is primarily social and daily living connections, but cognitive and motor skills play a part as well. These are activities that the participant can do alone, or in a group. Something as simple as greeting the dog allows the participant to make a connection, initiate conversation and reach out to the dog, demonstrating a degree of mobility. When the dog is close by, sometimes the basic need to care for others emerges, and a participant may willingly dress the dog, and in turn be encouraged to help themselves put on articles of clothing. Once the ball is rolling, it leads to so much more.

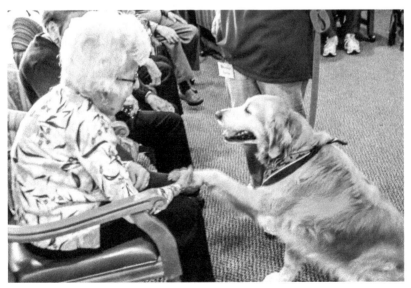

How do you do?

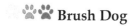 Brush Dog

Suitable Cognitive/Functional Impairment Level

Mild	Moderate	Severe

Connection:
Cognitive: Attention, Follow directions, Language, Numbers
Motor: Grasp objects, Hand-eye coordination, Manual dexterity, Range of motion
Social: Caring for others, Control, Initiate conversations, Staying calm

Equipment:
Dog brush or mitt

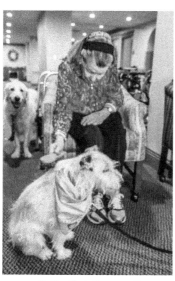

Rufus first, Izzy next!

Procedure:
Position dog in front of or next to participant.
Dog can sit, stand, or be in participant's lap.
Hand brush to participant.
Participant brushes dog.

> **Tip:** This activity can also encourage a person to comb or brush his/her own hair and focus on grooming. Counting brush strokes out loud encourages language as well as number sequencing.

Modification: Handler may need to assist in the brush holding, and may even have to assist with the brushing motion.

Crawl

Suitable Cognitive/Functional Impairment Level

Mild	Moderate	Severe

Connection:
Cognitive: Attention, Communication, Language
Motor: Balance, Range of motion, Upper body movement
Social: Cooperation, Eye contact, Self control

Equipment:
Treats

Procedure:
Position dog several feet away from participant.
Participant gives command "down."
Then, participant gives "crawl" command to dog.
Dog crawls to participant.
Participant gives dog a treat.

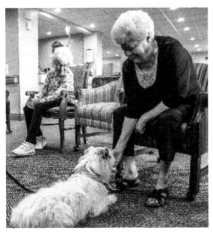

Modification:
Handler can give "crawl" command, if participant is unable.

Crawling to the treat

🐾 Doggie Doggie, Where's Your Bone?

Suitable Cognitive/Functional Impairment Level

Mild	Moderate	Severe

Connection:
Cognitive: Language, Communication, Follow directions, Memory, Perception
Motor: Grasp objects, Manual dexterity
Social: Asking questions, Cooperation, Eye contact, Teamwork

Equipment:
Treats

Procedure:
Participants sit in a circle.
Dog is positioned in center of circle.
Handler places blindfold on dog.
One participant is given a treat to hide in his/her hand.
All hold out closed fists, and chant,
      "Doggie doggie, where's your bone?"
Handler removes blindfold.
Handler leads dog around to each participant's outstretched fists to find the treat.

Modification:
For small groups, handler can work separately with each participant, and have them hide the treat in a hand, one by one. Dog chooses which hand the treat is in. Participant, opens hand, and gives the dog the treat.

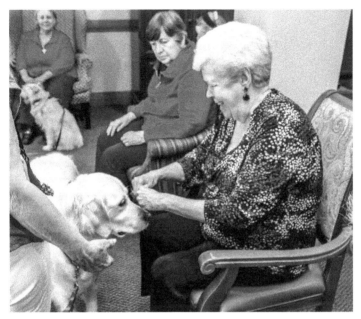

Doggie, doggie, where's your bone?

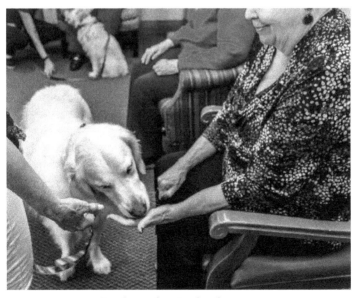

Izzy knows how to play the game.

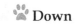 Down

Suitable Cognitive/Functional Impairment Level

Mild	Moderate	Severe

Connection:
Cognitive: Attention, Communication, Language, Perception
Motor: Balance, Manual dexterity, Range of motion, Upper body movement
Social: Cooperation, Eye contact

Equipment:
Treats

Procedure:
Position dog facing the participant.
Participant gives the command "down."
Dog "downs."
Participant gives dog a treat.

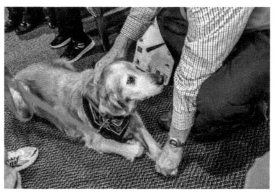
Good "down"

Modifications:
Handler can give hand signal for down so that the dog appears to be listening to the participant, if the verbal command is soft.

Dressing

Suitable Cognitive/Functional Impairment Level

Mild	Moderate	Severe

Connection:
Cognitive: Attention, Follow directions, Language, Reasoning, Sequencing, Visual and spatial processing
Motor: Grasp objects, Hand-eye coordination Manual dexterity
Social: Control, Cooperation, Caring for others, Eye contact

Equipment:
Dog clothing (bandana, sweater, vest, scarf)
People Clothing (hat, gloves, vest)

Procedure:
Position dog in front of participant.
Ask participant to help dress the dog.
Then suggest that participant take a turn.
Participant can put on gloves, hat, etc.
Tell dog to "take it."
Dog removes or brings hat, gloves, etc.
Activity can be repeated.

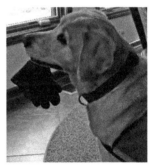
Brightie brings gloves

Tip: Good opportunity for caregiver participation. Motivation for dressing, by involving the dog getting dressed as well. A conversation starter for topics such as seasons, appropriate dress.

Modification:
"Dress yourself." Assist participant, with the goal of having the participant "dress" as independently as possible.

Putting on slippers:
Place slippers several feet from participant.
Participant tells dog, "bring my slippers" (or other command such as "get it" or "take it").
Dog brings slippers (one at a time).
Participant puts slippers on.
Participant asks dog to take slippers off (one at a time).
Dog hands each slipper to participant.
Can do the same with gloves or a hat instead of slippers.

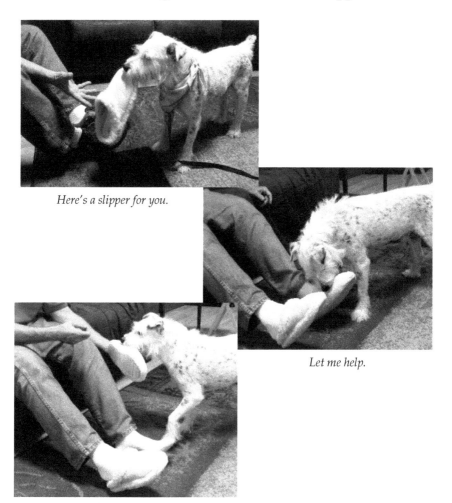

Here's a slipper for you.

Let me help.

Here you go!

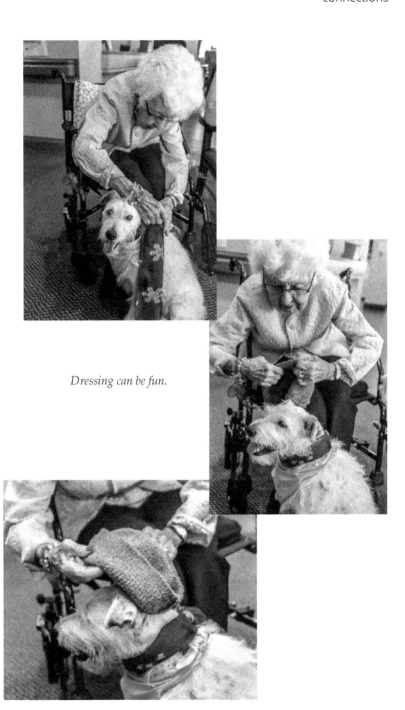

Dressing can be fun.

🐾 Give a dog a drink

Suitable Cognitive/Functional Impairment Level

Mild	Moderate	Severe

Connection:
Cognitive: Attention, Follow directions, Language, Perception, Reasoning, Sequencing
Motor: Grasp object, Manual dexterity, Range of motion
Social: Caring for others, Cooperation, Feeding, Teamwork

Equipment:
Water bottle
Dog bowl

Procedure:
Position dog in front of or next to participant.
Participant unscrews cap from water bottle, and pours water into the dog's bowl (bowl can either be on the floor or held by the handler).
Participant can tell the dog, "have a drink."

Modification:
Handler can assist with opening the water bottle, and pouring the water into the bowl.

Tip: This can be a cooperative effort, with one participant opening the water, another pouring, and another giving the dog a drink.

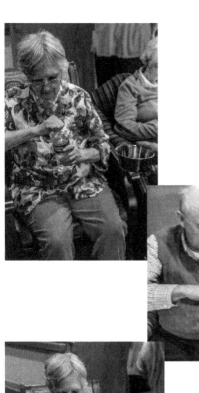

Cooperation and assistance

Zoe appreciates the team effort.

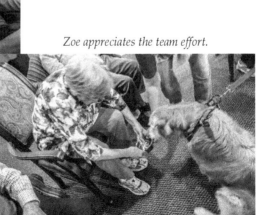

🐾 Give Tissue

Suitable Cognitive/Functional Impairment Level

Mild	Moderate	Severe

Connection:
Cognitive: Attention, Follow directions, Language
Motor: Grasp objects, Hand-eye coordination, Manual dexterity
Social: Cooperation, through interaction with dog

Equipment:
Box of tissues

Procedure:
Position dog in front of or next to participant.
Place box of tissues within reach of the dog.
Participant pretends to sneeze.
Dog hands tissue to participant.
Participant gives dog a treat.

Modification:
Handler pretends to sneeze.
Dog hands tissue to handler.

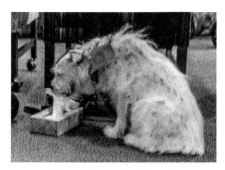

Okay, who needs a tissue?

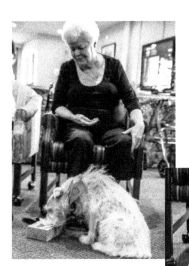

Achoo!!

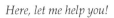

Here, let me help you!

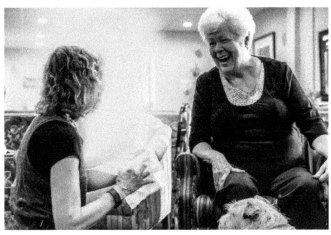

Rufus is good help, and good entertainment!

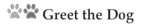 Greet the Dog

Suitable Cognitive/Functional Impairment Level

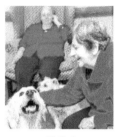

Mild	Moderate	Severe

Hello!

Connection:

Cognitive: Attention, Communication, Language, Perception

Motor: Hand-eye coordination, Manual dexterity, Range of motion

Social: Asking questions, Expressing feelings, Eye contact. Meeting, Greeting, Initiate conversation

Equipment:

Treats

Procedure:

Position dog in front of participant.

Ask if participant would like to pet the dog, shake his hand, give him a high five, etc.

Have participant give dog a treat.

Tip: As the dog visits each participant, conversation and communication is encouraged not only with the dog, but among other participants.

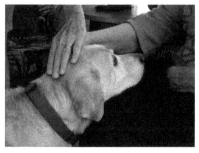

Greeting Brightie with assistance

Modification:

If the participant is severely impaired, a family member or staff member could place the participant's hand on the dog, helping to pet.

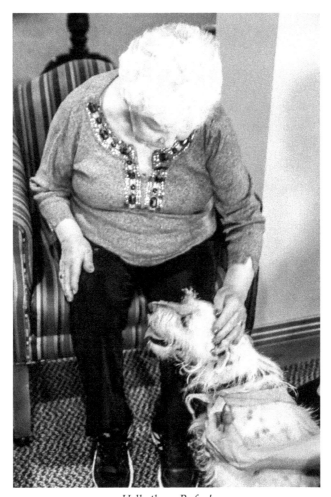

Hello there, Rufus!

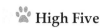 **High Five**

Suitable Cognitive/Functional Impairment Level

Mild	Moderate	Severe

Connection:
Cognitive: Attention, Follow directions, Language
Motor: Hand-eye coordination, Manual dexterity, Range of motion
Social: Asking questions, Eye contact, Cooperation, Initiate conversation, Meeting, Greeting

Equipment:
Treats
Gloves

Procedure:
Position dog sitting, facing participant.
Participant gives the command "high five" while raising hand above the dog.
Dog raises paw to touch participant's hand with a "high five."

Modification:
Handler can give the dog a high five, if participant is unable.

Tip: A glove can be used on the participant's hand, to prevent scratching delicate skin.

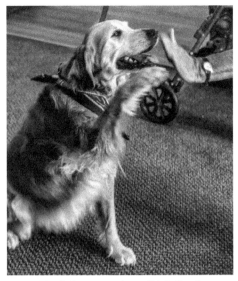

Zoe is happy to give a "high five."

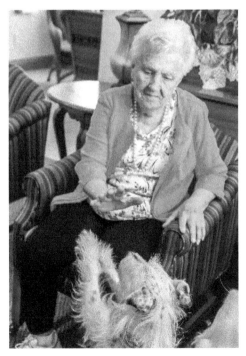

Rufus goes for the "high ten!"

🐾 Roll Over

Suitable Cognitive/Functional Impairment Level

Mild	Moderate	Severe

Connection:
Cognitive: Attention, Communication, Language,
Motor: Manual dexterity, Range of motion, Upper body movement
Social: Eye contact, Control, Cooperation

Equipment:
Treats

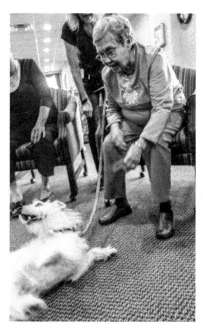

Rufus is on a "roll."

Procedure:
Position dog facing participant.
Participant gives command to "roll over."
Dog rolls over.
Participant gives dog a treat.

> **Tip:** Participant can be shown a hand signal to accompany the verbal command.

Modification:
If participant in unable to give hand signal, the handler can give it as the verbal command is given.

Shake

Suitable Cognitive/Functional Impairment Level

Mild	Moderate	Severe

Connection:
Cognitive: Attention, Follow directions, Language
Motor: Grasp objects, Manual dexterity, Range of motion
Social: Expressing feelings, Eye contact, Meeting, Greeting, Initiate conversations

Equipment:
Treats
Gloves

Procedure:
Position dog sitting, in front of participant.
Ask participant to give the command "shake," or "give paw," or whatever your dog's command is for this skill.
Dog lifts paw to "shake."

> **Tip:** Any time the dog's paw makes contact with the participant, a glove can be used to protect older, fragile skin.

Modification:
Handler can give the command to the dog, if participant is unable.

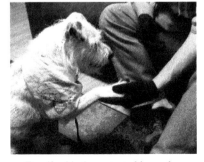

Fragile skin is protected by a glove.

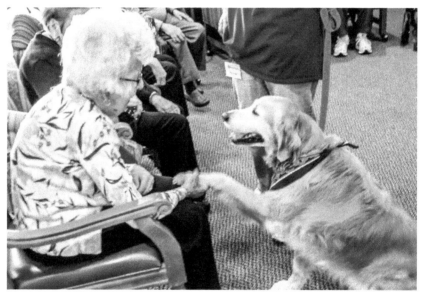

Making friends

Sit up

Suitable Cognitive/Functional Impairment Level

Mild	Moderate	Severe

Connection:
Cognitive: Attention, Communication, Language
Motor: Grasp objects, Manual dexterity
Social: Cooperation, Eye contact, Staying calm

Equipment:
Treats

Procedure:
Dog sits and faces participant.
Participant tells the dog to "sit up."
Dog sits up.
Participant gives dog a treat.

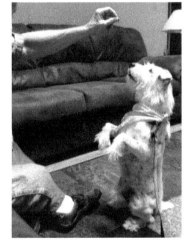

Focused!

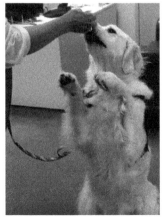

Modification:
Handler can give the dog the treat, if participant is unable.

Izzy sits pretty.

95

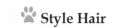 **Style Hair**

Suitable Cognitive/Functional Impairment Level

Mild	Moderate	Severe

Connection:
Cognitive: Attention, Follow directions, Language, Sequencing, Visual and spatial processing
Motor: Balance, Grasp objects, Manual dexterity, Range of motion
Social: Caring for others, Control, Cooperation, Initiate conversations, Staying calm

Equipment:
Dog brush
Hair accessories suitable for dog's hair (barrettes, scrunchies, etc.)

Procedure:
Position dog in front of or next to participant.
Demonstrate how to apply hair accessories to the dog's fur.
Participant chooses accessories to apply to dog.

> Tip: Be creative, be silly, have fun!

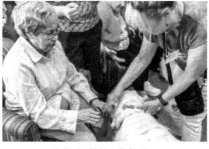

A little "bling" for Izzy

Modification: If manual dexterity is limited, the participant can give directions to handler on how to "accessorize." The handler can also offer a guiding hand to participant.

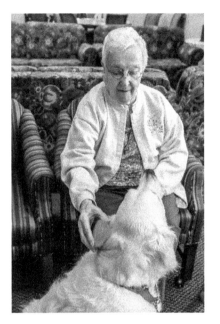

Prepare to style.

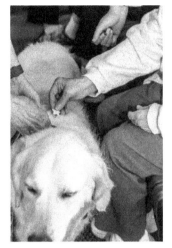

Place the clips.

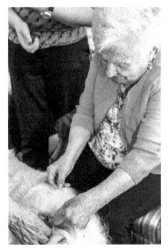

Place the clips with assistance.

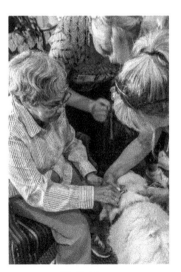

Stylin' Izzy.

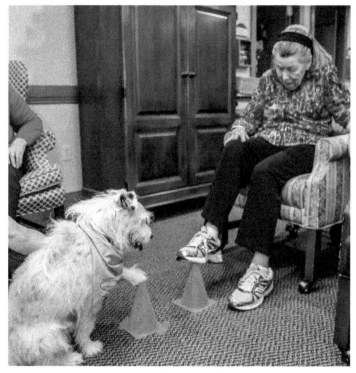

Workin' out!

11

Motor Skills, Physical Connections

The primary focus of the activities in this chapter is motor skills, both large and small. By virtue of participating in these activities, social and cognitive skills are naturally integrated. Taking a walk triggers conversation, and a concentration on the dog at the end of the leash. Just kicking a soccer ball around encourages language and a thought process about where to direct the kick. Hands can easily grasp rings for a ring toss game, or can grasp any number of objects involved with these activities.

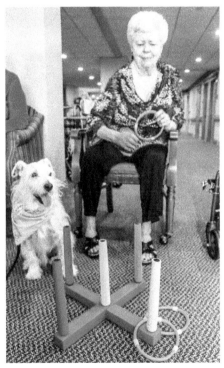

Movement, Concentration, Perception

🐾 Basketball

Suitable Cognitive/Functional Impairment Level

Mild	Moderate	Severe

Connection:
Cognitive: Attention, Perception, Visual and spatial processing
Motor: Grasp objects, Manual dexterity, Hand-eye coordination, Range of motion
Social: Control, Cooperation, Teamwork

Equipment:
Small hand held basketball hoop
Small ball (I use a rubber ball that looks like a small basketball!)

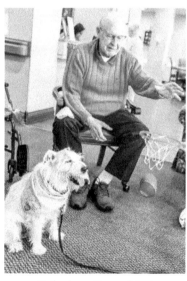

Rufus is pretty confident he can get the rebound.

Procedure:
Position dog facing, or next to participant.
Hand the ball to participant.
Hold the hoop out in front of participant.
Ask participant to toss the ball into the hoop.
Whether or not a basket is made, the dog can pick up the "rebound" and bring the ball back and drop it in the hoop.

Modification:
Participant can hold the hoop (with assistance if necessary) for the dog.

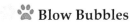 Blow Bubbles

Suitable Cognitive/Functional Impairment Level

Mild	Moderate	Severe

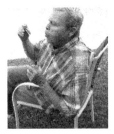

Concentration

Connection:

Cognitive: Attention, Follow directions, Language, Visual and spatial processing

Motor: Grasp objects, Manual dexterity, breath control

Social: Cooperation, teamwork, encourage laughter, emotion

Equipment:
Doggie bubbles

Tip: There are edible, dog friendly bubbles available at pet specialty shops.

Procedure:
Position dog facing or next to participant.
Handler gives bubbles to participant.
Participant blows bubbles.
Dog catches, breaks bubbles.

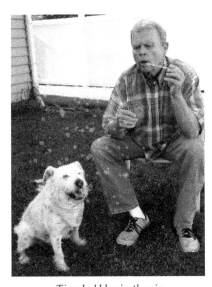

Modification:
Handler can hold bubbles and wand for participant.
Handler encourages participant to "blow."

Tiny bubbles in the air

Bow

Suitable Cognitive/Functional Impairment Level

Mild	Moderate	Severe

Connection:
Cognitive: Attention, Language, Perception
Motor: Balance, Mobility, Range of motion, Upper body movement
Social: Cooperation, Eye contact, Meeting, Greeting, Initiate conversation

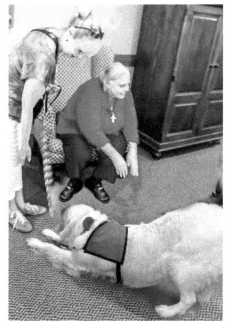

Take a bow.

Equipment needed:
Treats

Procedure:
Position dog facing the participant.
Participant gives command to "bow."
Participant bows with the dog.

Tip: After any activity, the dog can take a bow. Participant can bow back! Or the bow can be used as a greeting.

Modification: The handler can tell the dog to "bow" verbally or with a hand signal.

Bowling

Suitable Cognitive/Functional Impairment Level

Mild	Moderate	Severe

Connection:
Cognitive: Attention, Follow directions, Language, Numbers, Perception, Sequencing, Visual and spatial processing
Motor: Balance, Grasp objects, Hand-eye coordination, Mobility, Range of motion
Social: Control, Cooperation, Teamwork

Equipment:
Bowling pins (could be lightweight plastic toy pins, or sections of Styrofoam "noodles")
Bowling ball (lightweight ball, nerf-like)
Tray or mat for setting up pins

Procedure:
Position dog next to participant.
Handler sets up bowling pins on a tray or a mat.
Participant rolls ball toward pins.
Participant counts how many are knocked over.
Pins are "re-set."
Then, participant hides treat between pins (pins can be brought to participant on tray, then set on floor).
Participant tells dog to "go bowling."
Dog finds treat among the pins, participant counts how many pins are knocked down.
Score can be kept for participant and dog.

Modification:
Handler can hide treat by the pins if participant is unable.

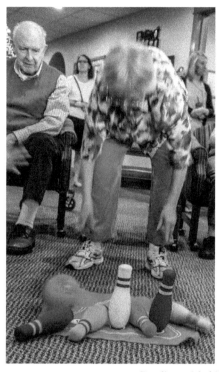

Bowling with friends.

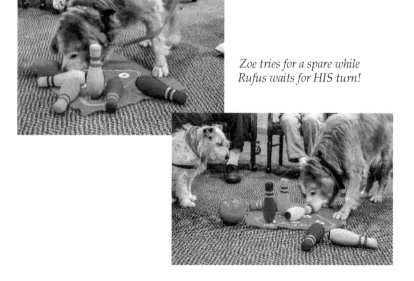

Zoe tries for a spare while Rufus waits for HIS turn!

Buzzers

Suitable Cognitive/Functional Impairment Level

Mild	Moderate	Severe

Connection:
Cognitive: Colors, Follow directions, Language, Sorting
Motor: Upper body, Range of motion, Hand-eye coordination
Social: Cooperation, Initiate conversation, Teamwork

Equipment:
Variety of buzzers

Procedure:
Position dog facing participant.
Place buzzrs on table or floor between dog and participant.
Participant chooses buzzer by color or shape.
Participant tells dog to "buzz" it.

Modification: Participants can try out the buzzers first.

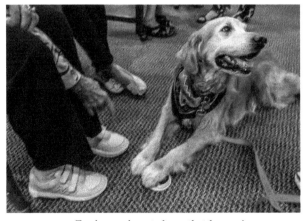

Zoe knows how to buzz that buzzer!

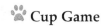 Cup Game

Suitable Cognitive/Functional Impairment Level

Mild	Moderate	Severe

Connection:
Cognitive: Attention, Colors, Language, Memory, Reasoning, Visual and spatial processing
Motor: Grasp objects, Hand-eye coordination, Manual dexterity
Social: Cooperation, teamwork

Equipment:
Three different colored cups
Tray for cups
Bandana-blindfold for dog
Treats

Procedure:
Place blindfold on dog. Or position dog facing away from participant, so dog can't "peek."
Ask participant to place a treat under one of the cups.
Participant can "mix up" the cups.
Participant removes bandana, or handler turns dog to face participant.
Participant tells dog to "find it."

Modification:
Use a muffin tin with tennis balls. If the participant is unable to hide the treat under the cup, this is an easier way for a participant to drop a treat (or two!) in the muffin tin, then place balls over the cups.

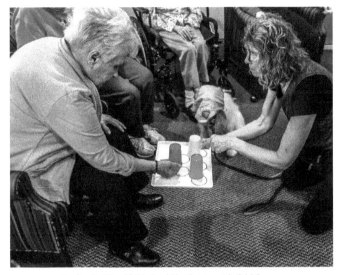

Rufus is blindfolded while the treat is hidden.

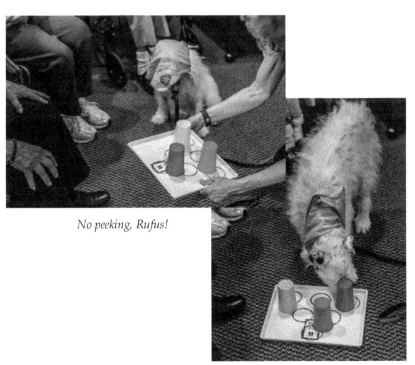

No peeking, Rufus!

Rufus searches for the treat.

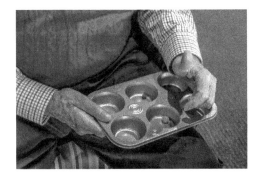

*The modification:
Treats in a muffin tin hidden
by tennis balls*

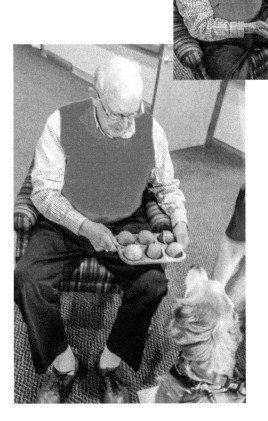

*A double win for
Zoe…tennis balls
AND treats!*

Dance

Suitable Cognitive/Functional Impairment Level

Mild	Moderate	Severe

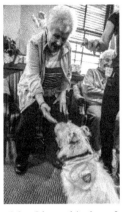

May I have this dance?

Connection:
Cognitive: Attention, Language, Memory, Perception
Motor: Balance, Range of motion, Mobility
Social: Cooperation, Control, Eye contact, Initiate conversation

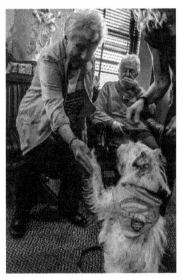

Doin' the jive!

Equipment:
Treats
Music (optional)

Procedure:
Participant gives command to dog to dance and holds a treat above dog's head.
Participant makes a circular motion with arm and hand as the command "dance" is verbalized.

Modification: Handler can give the "dance" command, and the participant, if able, can stand and dance alongside the dog.

🐾 Leg lifts with Cone

Suitable Cognitive/Functional Impairment Level

Mild	Moderate	Severe

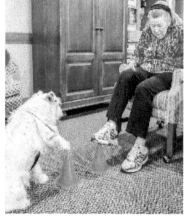

Rufus matches the move.

Connection:
Cognitive: Attention, Language, Memory, Numbers, Sequencing Visual and spatial processing
Motor: Balance, Range of motion
Social: Cooperation, eye contact

Equipment:
Plastic cones

Procedure:
Position dog, sitting, facing participant. Place one cone in front of the dog, the other cone in front of participant, a "leg length" away.

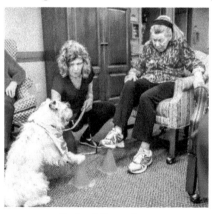

Rufus follows along.

Participant is told to raise one leg, placing heel on the cone, then to remove foot from cone. Participant is told to raise the other leg, placing that heel on the cone, then to remove it Continue, alternating legs. Meanwhile, the dog follows along with the participant, alternating front paws on the cone.

Modification: Encourage language by asking participant to say "right, left, right, etc." Or, participant can count the number of times the cone is touched.

🐾 Marching in Place

Suitable Cognitive/Functional Impairment Level

Mild	Moderate	Severe

Connection:
Cognitive: Attention, Follow directions, Language, Memory, Sequencing
Motor: Mobility, Range of motion
Social: Cooperation, Eye contact, Teamwork

Equipment:
Chair

Procedure:
Position dog facing participant.
Participant is sitting in a chair.
Leader gives direction to lift one leg, then the other, marching in place.
Dog alternately lifts paws with participant.

March right...

> Tip: Encourage language as each foot is lifted, by telling the dog "March right, March left." Or, by counting the steps out loud.

Modification:
Dog can be positioned closer to participant, and as each foot is lifted, the dog touches his paw on the participant's foot.

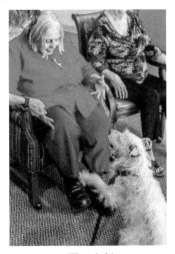

Then left!

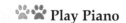 **Play Piano**

Suitable Cognitive/Functional Impairment Level

Mild	Moderate	Severe

Connection:
Cognitive: Attention, Colors, Language, Memory, Sequencing
Motor: Hand-eye coordination, Manual dexterity
Social: Cooperaton, Teamwork

Equipment:
Toy Piano

Procedure:
Handler shows, demonstrates the piano to participant.
Handler asks if participant would like to play it.
Participant plays piano.
Ask participant if he/she thinks the dog can play it.
Place piano on floor.
Participant tells dog to "play it."
Participant can take turns with the dog playing the piano.

Tip: Any type of toy piano may be used, as well as any size.

Modification:
Handler can assist participant in "playing" piano.
Order can be reversed, so that dog can play it first, which may encourage participant to respond to the sound, then take a turn.

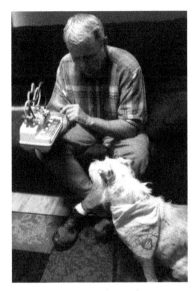

A song for Rufus

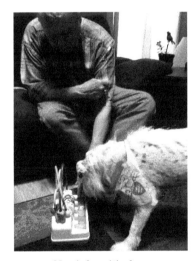

Here's how it's done.

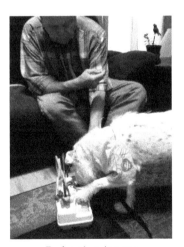

Rufus gives it a try.

🐾 Play Tambourine

Suitable Cognitive/Functional Impairment Level

Mild	Moderate	Severe

Connection:
Cognitive: Attention, Language, Perception, Sequencing
Motor: Manual dexterity, Hand-eye coordination
Social: Cooperation

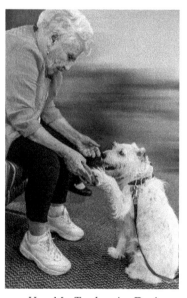

Equipment:
Tambourine

Procedure:
Position dog in front of participant.
Participant holds tambourine.
Participant taps tambourine.
Participant holds tambourine out to dog and gives the command to "play it."
Dog touches with paw.

Hey, Mr. Tambourine Dog!

Modification:
Handler can hold tambourine for participant to "play it."
Then, handler can hold tambourine for the dog.

Puzzle

Suitable Cognitive/Functional Impairment Level

Mild	Moderate	Severe

Connection:
Cognitive: Attention, Language, Memory, Numbers, Perception, Reasoning, Visual and spatial processing
Motor: Grasp objects, Hand-eye coordination, Manual dexterity
Social: Cooperation, Teamwork

Equipment:
Bandana for dog blindfold
Dog puzzle
Treats

Procedure:
Position dog in front of participant.
Place blindfold on dog.
Or, position dog facing away from participant, so dog can't "peek."
Participant hides treats in puzzle.
Participant removes bandana, or handler turns dog to face participant.
Participant tells dog to "find it."

Modification:
Handler can assist with removing bandana. Can be played in a group, with one person placing blindfold on dog, the other hiding the treats. Involve other participants by having another person remove the blindfold, and say "find it."
The participant can count out loud how many treats are being hidden. Then, as the dog finds the treats, they can be counted. The entire group can count along.

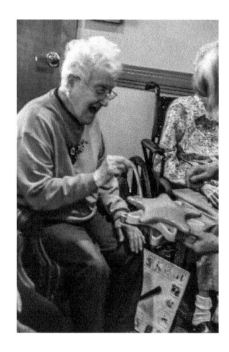

*Hiding the treats
in two different puzzles.*

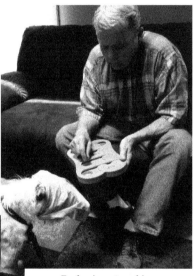

Rufus is not peeking.

*Rufus tries to find
every last treat.*

⁂ Ring Bell

Suitable Cognitive/Functional Impairment Level

Mild	Moderate	Severe

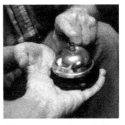

Participant rings bell.

Connection:
Cognitive: Attention, Language, Perception
Motor: Hand-eye coordination, Manual dexterity
Social: Cooperation

Equipment:
Bell, various types

Procedure:
Position dog facing participant.
Bell is placed on floor.
Participant tells dog to "ring it."
Dog rings the bell.
Bell is placed in front of participant.
Participant rings bell.

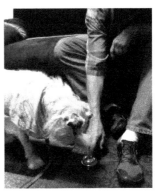

Rufus follows directions.

Modification: Use different types of bells.

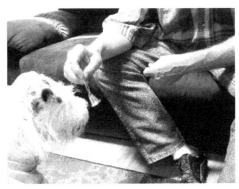

Rufus puts his nose to work.

117

🐾 Ring Toss

Suitable Cognitive/Functional Impairment Level

Mild	Moderate	Severe

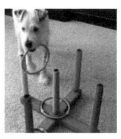

Taking a turn

Connection:

Cognitive: Attention, Colors, Follow directions, Language, Numbers, Perception

Motor: Grasp objects, Manual dexterity, Hand-eye coordination, Range of motion

Social: Cooperation, Initiate conversation, Teamwork

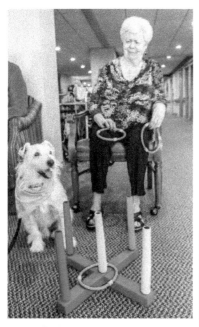

Rufus is ready to retrieve rings.

Equipment:
Ring toss game, or cones with other rings

Procedure:
Position dog next to participant.
Hand rings to participant.
Participant tosses the rings onto the game or cones.
Dog retrieves rings and hands them back to participant.

Tip: Various colors of rings may be used. Participants can count how many are thrown and/or reach the target. Create your own variations!

Modification: Dog can take a turn by fetching rings for participant, then putting rings onto the game.

Soccer

Suitable Cognitive/Functional Impairment Level

Mild	Moderate	Severe

Connection:
Cognitive: Follow directions, Attention, Language, Perception
Motor: Range of motion, Lower body
Social: Cooperation, Teamwork

Equipment:
Soft, lightweight medium to small ball

Procedure:
Participants are seated in a circle.
Position dog either in the center or next to one of the participants.
Ball is kicked to the center, or to another participant.
Or ball is kicked to the dog.
Dog picks up ball and brings it back to participant.

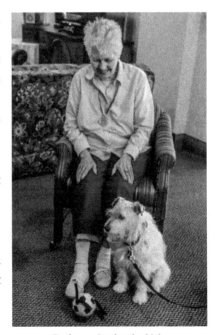

Modification: Handler can take turns with participant kicking the ball.

Rufus waits for the kick.

🐾 Stretching, Balance

Suitable Cognitive/Functional Impairment Level

Mild	Moderate	Severe

Connection:
Cognitive: Attention, Language, Perception
Motor: Balance, Hand-eye coordination, Range of motion, Upper body movement
Social: Cooperation, Initiate conversation

Equipment:
Chair

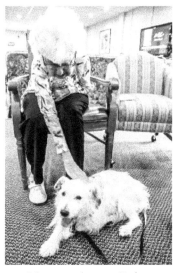

It's a stretch to pet Rufus.

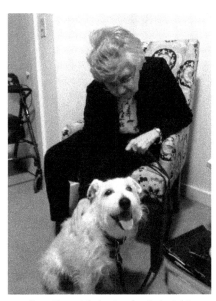

Sometimes it's just a short stretch!

Procedure:
Position dog sitting or lying down in front of participant. Participant is sitting in a chair. Participant stretches with both hands to pet dog. Then, position dog on one side. Participant reaches down on that side to pet the dog. Repeat for other side.

Modification:
Handler can assist as participant reaches down

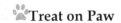
Treat on Paw

Suitable Cognitive/Functional Impairment Level

Mild	Moderate	Severe

Connection:
Cognitive: Attention, Perception, Language
Motor: Balance, Grasp objects, Hand-eye coordination, Manual dexterity, Range of motion
Social: Control, Cooperation, Staying calm

Equipment:
Treat

Procedure:
Position dog facing or next to participant.
Participant gives the "down" command.
Participant reaches down and places treat on dog's paw.
Participant gives "leave it" or "wait" command.
Wait several seconds.
Participant tells dog "okay."
Dog gets treat from paw.

> Tip: Participant can count out loud "one, two, three" before the okay command is given.

Modification:
If participant is unable to stretch down and put treat on paw, the participant can do the verbal commands, and handler can put treat on paw.

121

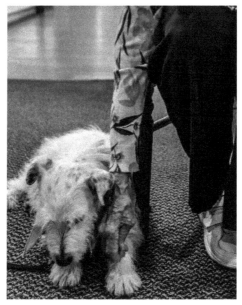

Reaching to place treat on paw

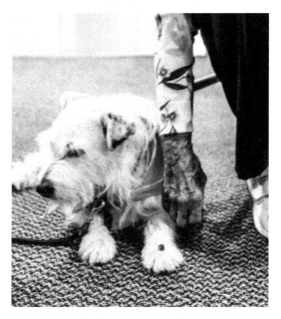

Rufus waits for the "okay."

🐾 Walk the Dog
Suitable Cognitive/Functional Impairment Level

Mild	Moderate	Severe

Connection:

Cognitive: Language, Visual and spatial processing, Sequencing
Motor: Gait skills, Balance, Wheel chair skills, Mobility, Motor planning
Social: Cooperation through interaction with dog, Control, Expressing feelings

Equipment:
Extra leash

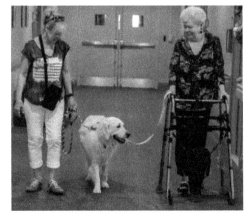

Zoe encourages walking.

Procedure:
Attach both leashes to dog's collar
Give one to participant to hold, keep the other.
Participant can either walk independently, with a walker or be in a wheelchair.
Dog walks alongside participant

Modification:
If participant has a walker, the second leash can be draped loosely on the walker. Participant can put hand over it.

Izzy makes sure her friend is walking alongside..

The Connectors

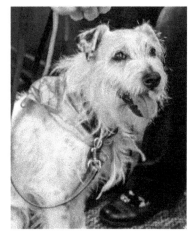

Rufus

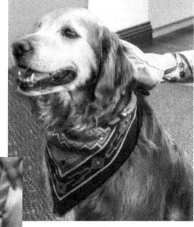

Zoe

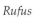

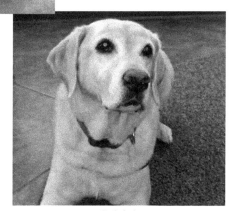

Izzy

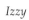

Brightie

EPILOGUE

It's now been over a year since I lost Mom. Rufus and I continue to visit the residents at Abbey Lane, where I still feel a connection to her. Little reminders of her still remain; in one of the living areas, a painting that she loved hangs on the wall, and her special Virgin Mary statue watches over the area.

Before her illness, Mom took great pride in looking good, having the right clothes, make-up, and hair done. The staff at Abbey Lane made sure that she was coordinated, right down to her jewelry. I became her "hairdresser" and made sure that she looked like the Irene we all knew. I would style her hair, and when I was done, I'd bring the mirror over and tell her that she looked "simply mahvelous, dahling." She would smile, and say it looked good. I always hoped that she knew it was her looking back at her.

But, it was not always about her looks. She led by example in so many other ways. As I was growing up, our home was always open to friends and family, and it wasn't unusual for us to wake up in the morning and find someone sleeping on our sofa who might be staying indefinitely. I wouldn't think twice about bringing home a friend or two for dinner. Somehow, there was always enough, and she would always insist that our guests take home any leftovers.

At Villa St. Benedict, there is a walkway with personalized memorial bricks, connecting two buildings. Rufus and I walk there before or after our visits, and we always stop for a while by one very special brick. It simply reads: "Irene Skwira, Family and Friends Always Welcome." That, I believe, says it all.

Dad has been gone for almost three years, but he left a legacy of compassion and caring. He exhibited extraordinary strength and dignity while caring for Mom all those years. During the last painful week of his life, whenever I was with him, and introduced him to any of the hospital staff, he would still lift his arm for that firm handshake he taught us and say, (though sometimes through gritted teeth) "It's a pleasure."

Rufus and I plan to continue our visits at least until he tells me he is ready to retire. Still on our docket are the hospital, library, and Abbey Lane. When we began as a therapy team, our focus was on children, but over the years, we have seen how Animal Assisted Therapy transcends all ages.

My journey with my parents blazed a trail for working with not only ADRD, but our aging population in general. For Rufus and me, this is another opportunity to make a difference, and continue making connections. Perhaps, through our work, we will be instrumental in the fight for Alzhheimer's first survivor.

Although Rufus will be thirteen this year, he shows no signs of slowing down. In addition to our visits, he is still always up for chasing a ball, catching a Frisbee, or licking a nose of someone he loves (or maybe someone he just met!).

I have experienced great joy from my partnership with Rufus. We always try to be prepared for our visits, taking pride in wearing our signature therapy vests, being well groomed, (Thanks, Mom!) and bringing appropriate equipment. And, when people thank us for visiting, I simply respond, "It's a pleasure." (Thanks, Dad!)

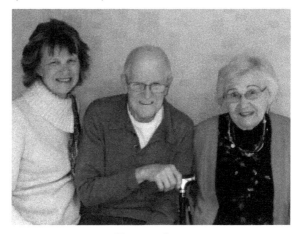

Always a pleasure

APPENDIX

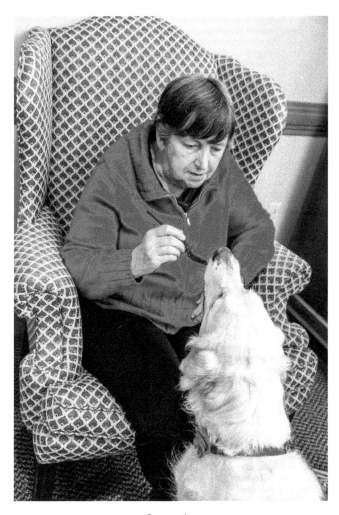

Connecting

10 Warning Signs of Alzheimer's Disease
Vs.
Typical Age Related changes

Alzheimer's	Typical age-related
1 Memory changes that disrupt daily life. Forgetting recently learned information or important dates.	Sometimes forgetting names, appointments, but remembering later.
2 Challenges in planning or solving problems. Trouble keeping track of bills, inability to develop and follow a plan.	Making occasional error when balancing checkbook.
3 Difficulty completing tasks at home, work or leisure. Such as remembering rules of a favorite game, managing a budget.	Occasionally needing help with settings on appliances.
4 Confusion with time or place. Lose track of dates, seasons, passage of time. May forget who they are how they got there.	Confused about day of the week, but remembering it later.
5 Trouble understanding visual images and spatial relationships. Difficulty reading, judging distance, perception, color contrasts.	Vision changes related to cataracts.

Alzheimer's	Typical age-related
6 New problems with words in speaking or writing. Hard to follow a conversation, stop in middle of conversation, cannot continue.	Sometimes having trouble finding the right word.
7 Misplacing things, losing ability to trace steps. Put things in unusual places. May accuse others of stealing.	Misplacing items from time to time, such as glasses or the remote control.
8 Decreased or poor judgment. With money, may give away large amounts to sales persons. Pay less attention to grooming, cleanliness.	Making a bad decision once in a while.
9 Withdrawal from work or social activities. May remove self from hobbies, social activities, work. May have trouble with a favorite hobby. Avoiding these activities.	Sometimes feeling weary of work, family and social obligations.
10 Changes in mood and personality. Become confused, suspicious, depressed, fearful, anxious.	Having a specific way of doing things and becoming irritable when the routine is disrupted.

(Basics of Alzheimer's. Alzheimer's Association)

Reisberg Functional Assessment Staging Scale (FAST)

Stage 1	Normal adult. No functional decline or difficulty.
Stage 2	Normal older adult. Personal awareness of forgetfulness, some functional decline.
Stage 3	Early Alzheimer's Deficits in demanding job functions..
Stage 4	Mild Alzheimer's. Assistance required with complex tasks such as handling finances, planning social events.
Stage 5	Moderate Alzheimer's. Assistance required with choosing proper clothing.
Stage 6	Moderately severe Alzheimer's. Assistance required with dressing bathing, toileting. Urinary and fecal incontinence.
Stage 7	Severe Alzheimer's. Declining loss of speech Decreased locomotion. Inability to smile, sit up, hold head up.

(www.dementiacarecentral.com)

Clinical Dementia Rating Scale (CDR)

CDR-0	No dementia.
CDR-0.5	Mild. Slight memory problems. Some difficulties with time and problem solving. Slight impairment in daily life.
CDR-1	Mild. Moderate memory loss with recent events, interfering with daily activities. Cannot function independently.
CDR-2	Moderate. Increased memory loss. Time and place disorientation. Impaired judgement. Decreased independence. Limited to simple chores.
CDR-3	Severe. Severe memory loss. Not oriented to time or place. Unable to participate in activities outside the home. Needs help with all tasks of daily living. Often incontinent.

(www.dementiacarecentral.com.)

Reisberg Global Deterioration Scale for Assessment of Primary Degnerative Dementia (GDS)

Stage 1	Normal function, mentally healthy.
Stage 2	Very mild cognitive decline. Normal forgetfulness with age.
Stage 3	Increased forgetfulness. May get lost, have trouble finding the right words.
Stage 4	Decreased memory. Inability to complete tasks, denial about symptoms.
Stage 5	Increased memory deficiencies, needing some assistance to complete daily activities such as dressing, bathing, preparing meals.
Stage 6	Increased assistance needed to carry out daily activities. Decreased ability to speak, personality changes, delusions, compulsions.
Stage 7	Severe cognitive decline, resulting in functional decline, requiring assistance with most activities.

(www.dementiacarecentral.com)

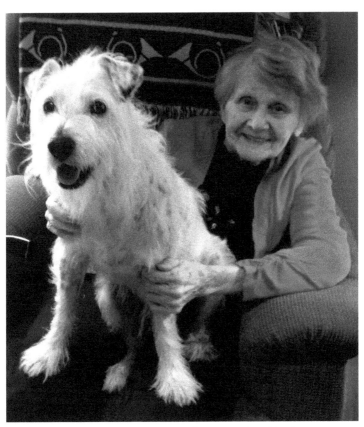

No matter where Mom sat, Rufus always found her lap.

Bibliography/Reference

Alzheimer's Disease and other Related Dementias

Books
Basics of Alzheimer's Disease. A Publication of the Alzheimer's Association.

Geriatrics at Your Fingertips, 2012 edition.
Reuben, David B., MD, et. al. American Geriatrics Society, New York, New York.

Learning to Speak Alzheimer's. Coste, Joanne Koenig 2003, Houghton Mifflin Company, New York.

Navigating Alzheimer's. Doyle, Mary K. 2015, In Extenso Press, Chicago, IL.

Online resources
www.alz.org. The Alzheimer's Association.

www.alzheimers.net. A Place for Mom.

www.americangeriatrics.org. The American Geriatrics Society.

www.caregiver.org. Family Caregiver Alliance.

www.dementiacarecentral.com. A wealth of information about Dementia, from types of Dementia to caregiver information.

www.ec-online.net. Eldercare online. Description of the FAST scale, and other helpful information.

www.mayoclinic.org/diseases-conditions/alzheimers-disease/in-depth/alzheimers-stages/art-20048448. Describes the Clinical dementia Rating Scale, and provides information about Dementia and Alzheimer's Disease.

Animal Assisted Therapy

Books
Animal Assisted Therapy Activities to Motivate and Inspire. Nancy Lind, 2009.

Animal Assisted Therapy: Techniques and Exercises for Dog Assisted Interventions. Francesc Ristol and Eva Domenec, 2012.

Teaming With Your Therapy Dog (New Directions in the Human-Animal Bond). Ann R. Howie, 2015.

101 Creative Ideas for Animal Assisted Therapy. Stacy Grover, 2010.

Online resources

https://www.1fur1.org/animal-assisted-therapy-improves-lives-helping-alzheimers-dementia-patients/
Animal Assisted Therapy Helps Alzheimer's and Dementia Patients.

http://blog.alz.org/tag/animal-assisted-therapy/

http://www.brightfocus.org/alzheimers/article/alzheimers-disease-magic-pets. Alzheimer's Disease, The Magic of Pets.

http://www.dogplay.com/Activities/Therapy/therapy1.html

www.everydayhealth.com. "How Animal Therapy Helps Dementia Patients," April 20, 2010, Madeline R. Vann, MPH. Medically Reviewed by Pat F. Bass, III, MD, MPH.

www.magonlinelibrary.com. "Animal Assisted Therapy for People Living with dementia," March 30, 2016, Aysha Mendes.

www.managedhealthcareconnect.com. "Animal Assisted Intervention Helps Patients with dementia," August 24, 2014, Leanne Taylor.

www.NIH.gov. "The Benefit of Pets and Animal Assisted Therapy to the Health of Older Individuals."

https://psychcentral.com/lib/the-truth-about-animal-assisted-therapy/. The Truth about Animal Assisted Therapy. Brandi-Ann Uyemura.

www.rover.com/canine-caregivers-dementia-alzheimers/ "The New Breed of Service Dog: Canine Caregivers for Dementia and Alzheimers Patients."

www.sciedu.ca/journal. (Journal of Nursing education and Practice) "Animal Assisted Therapy for Elderly Residents of a Skilled Nursing Facility," January 22, 2016, School of Nursing, Auburn University. William S. Pope, Caralise Hunt, Kathy Ellison.

www.travanseliving.com "Helping to Heal: The Benefits of Animal Assisted Therapy," October 14, 2016.

www.uofmhealth.org "How Therapy Animals Help Those Living with Dementia," June 8, 2016, Renee Gadwa.

https://www.verywell.com/how-does-pet-therapy-benefit-people-with-dementia-98677   How Does Pet Therapy Benefit People with Dementia. Esther Heerema, 2016.

Locate Therapy Dog groups in your area

www.landofpuregold.com.   (National organization).

https://petpartners.org/
Pet partners (National organization).

www.rainbowaat.org.   Rainbow Animal Assisted Therapy (Illinois-Chicago and suburbs organization).

http://www.tdi-dog.org/Introduction.aspx.
Therapy Dogs International (National organization).

https://www.therapydogs.com/.
Alliance of Therapy Dogs (National organization).

www.therapypets.com/jackies-list. (National listing).

Acknowledgements

This book is really about two journeys: the experience of working with a therapy dog, and the experience of having a loved one with Alzheimer's Disease and Related Dementias. Ten years ago, I'd been unaware that the two paths would cross

Whether it was the lives that Rufus and I touched over the years, or the people who touched our lives along our Alzheimer's journey, I am thankful to all of you.

To my friends at Rainbow Animal Assisted Therapy, especially Nancy Lind, who encouraged me and Rufus to return after that first training session! Rainbow's programs and support over the past 10 years have opened up a whole new world to me.

Our recent registration with the Alliance of Therapy Dogs allows Rufus and me to continue to visit Abbey Lane in an "official" capacity.

Villa St. Benedict is such an amazing place, and I am so happy that Mom was able to be a resident there. Thank you, staff and sisters, who truly live by the Benedictine Core Values of Hospitality, Respect, Stewardship, and Justice. I appreciate the sisters who stopped by to visit, and help Mom when she needed it.

From the moment we walked in to Villa St. Benedict, I felt we had a "home." And now, the support and cooperation of the entire community when Rufus and I visit, and during the course of writing this book, has been overwhelming.

Abbey Lane, the memory care unit where Mom lived, embodies all of those core values, and so much more. It has been said that a group's behavior is a reflection of its leadership, and

Kathy Fondriest is not only the head nurse of the area, but she led some wonderful support groups, along with colleague Heather Izumi. The two of them helped bring peace of mind to those of us struggling with loved ones affected by ADRD. Thank you both for your compassionate insight and knowledge.

In addition, Kathy Fondriest's professional suggestions and support during the creation of this book were invaluable.

I will never forget how Heather held my mom's hand until I could get to her, on the day that she died. You'll always have a special place in my heart for your kindness and caring. It's a privilege to count you among my friends.

I consider myself lucky to have been part of Villa St. Benedict's support group of children, spouses, or friends of loved ones with Dementia. Without it, I never would have met Donna Boughman and Ed Rog, who shared their personal journeys about their loved ones with Alzheimer's Disease. I found comfort and support hearing about so many surprisingly similar experiences. Out of that emerged wonderful friendships.

The nurses (especially Rose, who was with Mom during her last hours, making sure the polka music and sunshine surrounded her) and the CNA's always treated Mom as if she was their own Grandma. You are all top notch, in my estimation.

Thanks to Agnes Dzuibia for making sure that the residents were ready to visit with Rufus and the other teams. Your participation and support during our visits really enriched the experience for all.

A special thanks to the residents of Abbey Lane who demonstrated so much patience, compassion and understanding when Rufus and his friends visited. Not to mention how much fun you brought to our visits. You always made my day.

To the therapy teams of Jan Peterson and Zoe, Dee Thake and Izzy, and Jennifer Trojan and Brightie. Your patience and time really brought extra joy to the residents of Villa St. Benedict. You truly worked magic with your visits. Rufus especially appreciated his "girlfriends" taking over some of the activities!

Thank you to my friend, Marilyn Krelle, for sharing her photo of Rufus and me visiting her husband, Harvey at the hospital.

Tina Hussey, who with your mom, Mary Ellen, was always one step ahead of us in our journey with Alzheimer's Disease. You paved the way, and helped ease my concerns in so many ways by sharing your experiences and giving me your support and most importantly, friendship during such a tough, sometimes heartbreaking, time in our lives.

Carolyn Bartolotta, I am so fortunate to have your legal eagle eyes as part of this editing team. Your extensive experience with attention to detail is just what was needed.

Jari Lynn Franklin, I guess our high school yearbook editing partnership has come full circle. Your editing skills have not diminished over the years, much to my advantage.

Sally Woods, you are an author's dream editor. I am in awe of your serious editing expertise. I'm sure this is a better book as a result of your efforts.

Wayne Dunham, I sure appreciate you taking the time to contribute your thoughtful edits, despite juggling your own unbelievably frantic schedule.

Dulcey Lima, friend extraordinaire and award winning photographer, you are beyond exceptional. Thank you for spending time photographing the residents of Abbey Lane with our four legged therapists. You really captured their spirit. Sorting and editing the over 800 images, and whittling them down to what appears in the book was no small task. My gratitude is boundless.

To my brother, Al, who stayed on the same page with me during a wacky, stressful time of our lives. We each needed an ally, and there we were. I guess Mom and Dad did a good job!

My husband, Rick, who remained the even keel through this journey. You listened when I needed an ear, and gave me a shoulder to cry on. Then, you made me smile when you danced with Mom at Villa St. Benedict, and took the two of us to the Berwyn Moose for the dinner dance. A girl couldn't ask for more.

To my daughter, Kiki and my son, Cody, who, despite living on opposite coasts, always made time to visit Grandma and Grandpa when they came to town. You make me proud. Bringing Rufus into our lives that Christmas so many years ago turned out to be the ultimate gift that keeps on giving.

Cody, you took the time to go through the manuscript and bring me into the 21st century. Your photo editing expertise, cover design, and graphic creation are off the charts.

And finally, to Rufus, who has given me more that I can ever give him. He most generously gave me one-fourth of the office chair so that we could work together on this book.
What a dog.

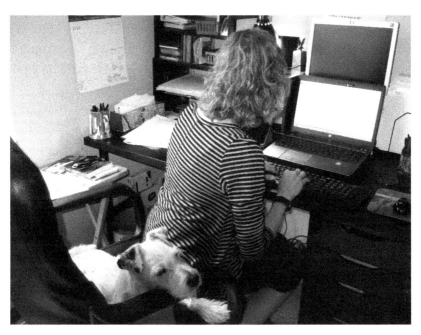

Rufus, ¾. Pam, ¼. As it should be

About the Author

Pam Osbourne is a writer and editor who has been involved in the publishing industry for over thirty years. She is a partner with Pull Your own Weight Publishing, a company through which she consults with authors who self-publish their own books. (pyowpublishing.webs.com)

She has worked in Animal Assisted Therapy programs with her Jack Russell Terrier, Rufus for over ten years. Together they have made a difference in the lives of people in schools, hospitals, libraries, and other settings in the western suburbs of Chicago.

She is an avid runner, having completed five marathons in recent years. She is also a weight lifter, which she says keeps her in shape for lifting Rufus.

CPSIA information can be obtained
at www.ICGtesting.com
Printed in the USA
LVHW01s1126160917
548787LV00002B/2/P